Painproof
How Habits Heal

Dr. Ariana Fontenot & Dr. Marla Lester
Doctors of Physical Therapy

Founders of The Slight Motion Method

Copyright © 2025
Painproof: How Habits Heal
[Ariana Fontenot & Marla Lester - Slight Motion PT]
All rights reserved. No part of this book may be reproduced, stored, or shared in any form without written permission from the author, except for brief excerpts used in reviews, educational content, or permitted by law.

Published by: Slight Motion PT / Self-Published via Amazon KDP

This book is for informational purposes only. It is not a substitute for professional medical advice, diagnosis, or treatment. Always consult a qualified healthcare provider for any medical concerns. The author and publisher disclaim any liability from the use or misuse of this book's content.

First Edition, 2025
Printed in the United States of America

www.slightmotionpt.com
Instagram @slightmotionpt
Email: slightmotionpt@gmail.com

Slight Motion Physical Therapy
"A Little Goes A Long Way"

Teamwork makes the dream work...

Without the incredible support and contributions of so many people, this book would not have been possible.

To our clients—you are the heart of this journey. It is an absolute privilege to help you heal, grow, and move toward a pain-free life. Your trust and dedication inspires everything we do.

To everyone who played a role in bringing this vision to life—your support, encouragement, and belief in this mission have fueled us every step of the way.

Together, we are changing lives and redefining what's possible—one person at a time.

Thank you for being part of this movement.

Table of Contents

How We Got Here 1
The Slight Motion Method 3
Pillow Talk 17
   Side Sleeping 20
   Back Sleeping 37
   Stomach Sleeping: Breaking the Habit 45
The Neck Chronicles 57
Wrist Whispers 91
Transportation Troubles 119
Shoulder Secrets 147
Thoracic Thoughts 171
Lumbar Lessons 189
Hip Habits 219
Knee Knowledge 247
Footwork Fundamentals 267
References 289
About The Authors 293
Testimonials 297

How We Got Here

The clinic was never quiet. Day after day, patients pushed through grueling sessions, believing that one hour of Physical Therapy could undo a lifetime of habits. They stretched, strengthened, and showed up week after week, trusting the system. But something didn't add up. They'd take 2 steps forward and 1 step back. They weren't getting better fast enough. They weren't maintaining their gains.

At first, I believed in the system too. I worked alongside my mentor and co-author, Dr. Marla Lester, refining techniques and delivering life-changing results. But as time went on, I saw the flaw: the system wasn't designed to heal people. It was designed to keep them coming back.

When I questioned that system, I became the problem.

I got fired…

For a moment, it felt like the end of the world. But in reality, I had just been set free.

Encouraged by my patients, I started treating people in their homes and workplaces—instead of in the clinic. That's when everything clicked.

Traditional Physical Therapy focused on one hour of their day, but the other 23 hours—filled with habits, postures, and movements—were silently reinforcing their pain.

A typical PT session was trying to undo in one hour what daily routines were constantly reinforcing. But pain doesn't start on a treatment table—it starts with the way people move every day. By stepping into my patients' real environments, I uncovered the true source of their pain—the hidden patterns that never surfaced in a clinic.

Dr. Lester and I began developing what is now known as the **Slight Motion Method**—an approach born from working with people where they live and move every day. Our work has consistently delivered results that far exceed the norm. In just one session, we've achieved breakthroughs that would typically take 20 visits in a clinic.

Referred to by many as the Rogue PT for rejecting the industry's playbook, I had discovered the truth: Pain isn't something you have to tolerate, it's something you can eliminate.

Instead of focusing on treating symptoms in isolation with unnecessary surgeries, medications, and injections, we've proven that addressing the root causes—the habits and environments that shape our daily lives—leads to faster, lasting results. Our patients aren't spending months in therapy. Instead, they're resolving their issues in just one or two sessions.

At its core, the **Slight Motion Method** is about empowering you to take control of your pain by addressing the little things that make the biggest difference.

This is more than a method—it's a movement.
And we can't wait for you to experience it.

Chapter 1
The Slight Motion Method

SLIGHT MOTION
Physical Therapy

"A Little Goes A Long Way"

What is the Common Theme in Each of These Photos?

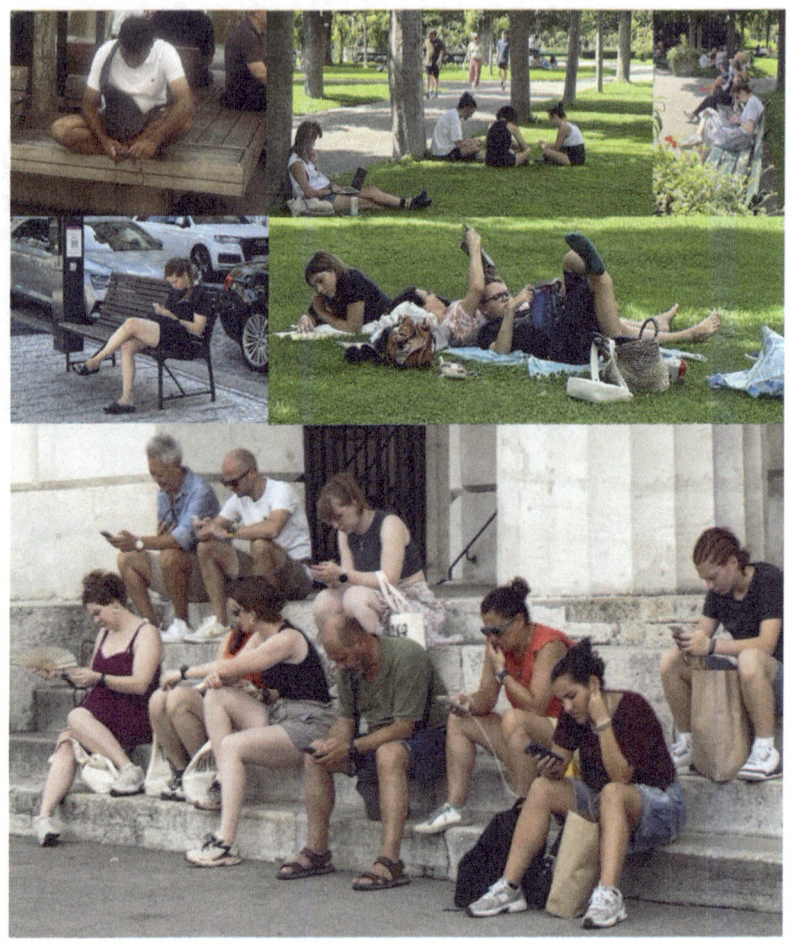

BAD POSTURE!

The Slight Motion Method

The essence of the **Slight Motion Method** is understanding that healing isn't about grand, dramatic interventions, but about the subtle, consistent changes we make every single day. It's about recognizing that our bodies are constantly speaking to us, and sometimes we just need to learn how to listen.

In traditional clinical settings, many of the cases you're about to read would have remained a medical mystery. Hour after hour of Doctor's appointments, countless medications, and years of temporary relief – all while missing the fundamental source of their pain.

A clinic can measure range of motion, provide exercises, and help you build strength and stability. But it can never truly understand the intricate landscape of a person's daily life. My approach is different. By stepping into my clients' homes, I become a detective of daily habits, uncovering the hidden triggers that perpetuate pain.

One client, Hope, was struggling with relentless migraines and jaw pain. No clinical assessment would have revealed the silent culprit. But in her bedroom, the cause became crystal clear—a seemingly minor detail in her sleep setup was subtly wreaking havoc on her body night after night. What looked like a simple pillow choice turned out to be the key to unlocking years of discomfort.

Hope's story is just one of many that reveal a fundamental truth: pain isn't always what it seems. It's not just about injuries or diagnoses—it's about patterns, habits, and environments.

In the pages ahead, you'll discover how small shifts in movement and daily routines can lead to profound, lasting change.

We don't just treat pain; we investigate its origin. Every home tells a story, and every room holds clues to understanding a person's physical challenges—kitchen counter too low, a chair without proper support, a sleeping position that causes full-body chaos. These are the root causes that traditional physical therapy in a clinic overlooks.

This is precisely why I reject the confines of a clinical environment and bring my practice directly into my clients' daily spaces.

In the rest of this book, we'll share everything we've learned with you. We're going to go from head to toe, learning how the things we do everyday affect each joint in our body. Our recommendation is to read one chapter a week and implement what you learn. Take note of how you feel after seven days. Apply what works for you, you'll be surprised how these seemingly little changes have a massive impact.

- Pillow Talk
- The Neck Chronicles
- Wrist Whispers
- Transportation Troubles
- Shoulder Secrets
- Thoracic Thoughts
- Lumbar Lessons
- Hip Habits
- Knee Knowledge
- Footwork Fundamentals

The House Call: Where Truth Reveals Itself

The beauty of Slight Motion PT is that we come to you! We are in your home, in your workplace, in the spaces you spend most of your day. We can trace the habits that directly correlate with your pain. There's a profound difference between what people tell you and what their environment reveals. I had a client who was convinced his chronic neck pain was from disc bulges, the result of a decade-old sports injury. Stepping foot into his home is where assumptions crumbled and the subtle truth emerged. His pillow, though seemingly positioned correctly, was nestled close enough to another pillow to create a slight tilt. Six hours of this subtle angle each night was enough to keep his neck in a perpetual state of strain.

When I showed him the photographs, his face lit up as if a hidden truth had just been uncovered. "I never even noticed," he admitted—a phrase I've heard countless times. But that's our job, to make you notice! We repositioned his pillow properly, ensuring there was no other pillow nearby to tilt it, and within weeks his pain was gone. Even a small shift in your pillow angle, like from a nearby pillow, can wreak havoc on your neck over time. This is why it's critical to evaluate your habits in your actual living environment. These subtle details often go unnoticed, but make all the difference.

The good news? The solution doesn't have to be as overwhelming as the problem. What if the secret to a pain-free life didn't require a drastic makeover? What if it came down to the little things you do every day? That's where the *Slight Motion Method* comes in.

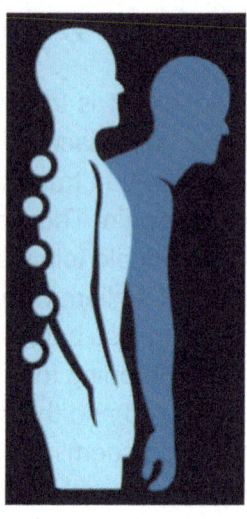

The *Slight Motion Method* was born from a simple yet profound realization: pain doesn't usually appear out of nowhere. Pain isn't just a feeling—it's a story, written every second by the little things we do (or don't do). It's our body's way of sending us a message. Muscle imbalances, strains, and postural tweaks accumulate over time, leaving us with discomfort we often accept as a normal part of aging and sometimes believe is permanent.

There is a common misconception that pain comes from a one time event that happened years ago, but pain doesn't have to be permanent. What if I told you that 2 minutes per day could change your life?

Our method is simple, yet influential. Small, intentional movements and changes in your daily habits can create a ripple effect, reshaping how your body feels and functions. These slight changes can dramatically reduce pain and prevent future injuries. It's not about marathon workouts, complicated routines, or massive lifestyle shifts.

If you're in pain and feel like you've tried everything, our goal is to introduce you to a method that transforms your daily habits and provide realistic solutions that fit seamlessly into your lifestyle—creating a lasting, lifelong impact on your well-being. When it comes to your body, a little truly goes a long way. No one is perfect, but we can always be better. Every small effort you make builds toward a better foundation.

Why the Little Things Matter

Many of the habits that contribute to our pain seem harmless at first. Looking down at your phone, your computer being at the wrong height, or spending hours on your couch every night watching TV may not feel painful in the moment, but over time, these little things add up.

I often think about how much we assume to be "common sense." Some things I'll never understand: why people don't wear their seatbelts, why they don't use their blinkers, or why they drive slowly in the passing lane. Maybe it's not that people ignore these rules—maybe they just don't know better.

The same applies to our bodies. I remember a friend who had hip surgery. Her post-surgical instructions were clear to us who are licensed Doctors of Physical Therapy: *toe-touch weight bearing only.* But would you know what that means? To her that meant she could tip-toe around as long as she didn't put any weight through her heels. What she didn't realize was that this was completely defeating the purpose of the precaution. It wasn't intentional—she just didn't know any better.

These seemingly small habits and misunderstandings can have big consequences, not because people don't care, but because they were never taught differently. For example how drinking out of a straw can cause stomach pain, or how taking pills without water can make acid reflux worse. Even something as simple as eating beets can leave people panicking—and sometimes rushing to the emergency room—when they mistake a harmless color change for a serious health issue, not realizing it's just the food they ate.

This book is about uncovering the little things we do every day and showing you how to make them healthier for your body. You'll learn about people just like you—individuals who were on the verge of seeking serious medical attention and found lasting relief through the **Slight Motion Method**, a game-changer when nothing else worked. Many experienced near-immediate relief, overcame their pain, and eliminated the need for surgery, injections, or other invasive treatments by addressing the root causes and preventing their pain from returning.

You don't need perfection. You just need small, intentional changes that work with your body, not against it. What if you could turn the habits you're already doing every day into exercise? By increasing your awareness and making your environment work for you instead of against you, you can create a foundation for lasting health and a pain-free life. With these tools, the things you already do every day can become the building blocks of a healthier, happier, and more sustainable lifestyle. A life that you love.

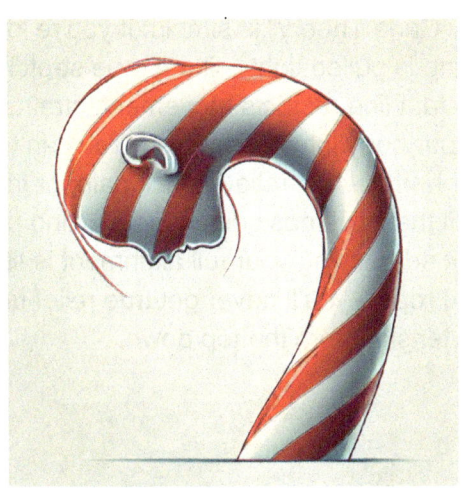

The Candy Cane Theory

The Candy Cane Theory reminds us that alignment isn't just about standing up straight—it's about honoring the invisible line that connects your body from head to toe. Imagine a rope running from your forehead to your toes. This line is the foundation of your body's alignment, the axis around which every movement, habit, and posture revolves. It should be balanced and free, but most of us unknowingly bend it into a candy cane—curved, strained, and tight. Trying to improve flexibility or strength with a curved candy cane is like building a house on a crooked foundation.

Every time you hunch over your phone, slump at your desk, or sleep in an awkward position, you reinforce that candy cane curve. Over time, this strain accumulates, creating tension and pain throughout your body.

The "Candy Cane Theory" is simple: if you're looking down, the line is pulled tight—like a rope stretched to its limit. A fully taut line restricts movement, strains muscles, and locks your body into dysfunction. You can't effectively stretch your hamstrings, relieve back pain, or improve mobility until that rope has some slack. Fixing pain in one area without addressing your full alignment is like tugging on a knotted rope—you'll never get true relief until you release the tension from the top down.

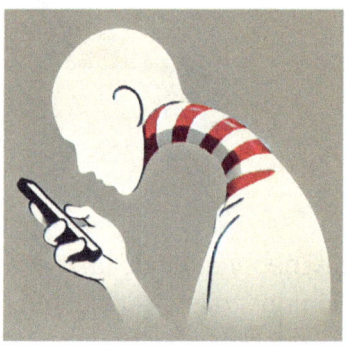

The goal isn't to correct the candy cane overnight, but to gradually guide your body back into alignment, one small change at a time. It might not be perfect, but it will be better! Aligning your foundation first ensures every movement builds strength and reduces pain. Start with the foundation, and the rest will take care of itself.

The mistake most people make? They try to undo 23 hours of bad habits with just 1 hour of exercise. But real change doesn't come from that single hour; it comes from what you do the rest of the day.

What if, instead of chasing perfection, you aimed for just 1% better each day? Small, consistent improvements add up. Start simple—would you be willing to hold a one-second plank every day? It sounds small, but that's the point. Consistency beats intensity when you're building lasting change.

But posture doesn't just affect your body—it shapes your mindset, too. When you look down, your body collapses inward, signaling stress, fatigue, and negativity. Look up, and everything shifts—your chest opens, your shoulders relax, and your brain receives a powerful cue of confidence and energy. Fixing your posture isn't just about avoiding pain—it's about feeling better in every way. The question is: are you reinforcing habits that pull you down, or creating alignment that lifts you up?

Building Your Body's Jenga Tower

Think of your spine like a Jenga tower—when it's stacked straight, it's stable and balanced. If past injuries or daily habits have shifted some of the blocks, it can create extra strain in certain areas. But unlike the game, your body is resilient and adaptable. This just means your habits need to support that resilience. You can't get away with things like slouching on the couch for hours or ignoring how you move. Small, consistent changes in your daily habits can keep your "tower" strong, stable, and pain-free.

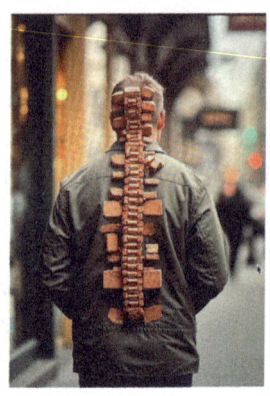

Understanding the Ripple Effect of Pain

Pain often feels random, but it's rarely without cause. The truth is, if you're having good days, you're probably the one creating your bad days. Pain doesn't always show up immediately; it's a lagging indicator. Just like when you work out, you're typically not sore the same day, but feel it 1-3 days later. Pain reflects what you did—or didn't do—several days ago.

For example, if it rains on a weekend and you spend hours on the couch in poor positions, you might feel fine at first. But by Tuesday or Wednesday, that discomfort you're feeling isn't a mystery, it's the result of those habits catching up to you.

Here's the challenge: when you're in pain, the natural instinct is to rest. While rest can feel like the right thing to do, it often compounds the problem. Why? Because most people rest in nonoptimal positions—slouched on the couch, curled up in bed, or hunched over their phones. These positions reinforce the very habits that contributed to the pain in the first place.

This is why awareness and prevention are critical. Pain is cumulative, and small changes today can prevent major setbacks tomorrow. The more intentional you are with your habits, the fewer "bad days" you'll have to endure.

Movement is Medicine

Your spine is like a tree. If you hit the same part of the tree over and over, eventually it will fall. But if you hit it a little higher or lower, it'll have time to repair and strengthen itself. The spine, much like a tree, is remarkably adaptable and self-sustaining.

This is the essence of why movement is medicine. By varying how you position yourself, you give your body the chance to adapt and grow stronger. If you repeatedly strain the same area of your body without addressing these patterns, pain becomes inevitable. But when you change even the smallest habits—like standing evenly on both feet, using an adjustable desk, using a rocking chair, or realigning your sitting posture—your body begins to heal itself naturally.

Breaking the Cycle

In our career, we've seen countless clients fall into the same trap. They visit clinics, massage therapists, or chiropractors searching for relief. While these treatments may bring short-term relief, they don't address the root of the problem. Why? Because if you go home and continue the same patterns that caused the pain in the first place, you'll never truly be "pain-free". What seems like common sense once it's pointed out, wasn't always so obvious, as these habits have become so routine.

By the end of this book, you'll understand how to "Painproof" your life and learn simple ways to implement these new habits into your current way of life. The slightest improvements can take away pain—and over time, those small changes will transform your life. It's not about the one hour you do or don't spend in the gym. This book is about the other 23 hours of the day that you can take advantage of.

You don't need to be perfect to feel better. You just need to start. Let's begin by uncovering the little things that make a big difference.

Let's start building a better foundation, one slight motion at a time.

Chapter 2
Pillow Talk

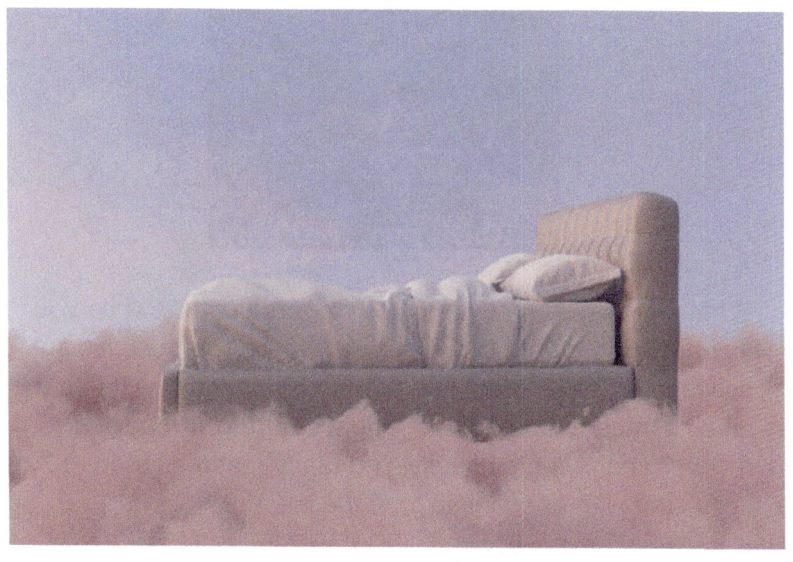

Pillow Talk

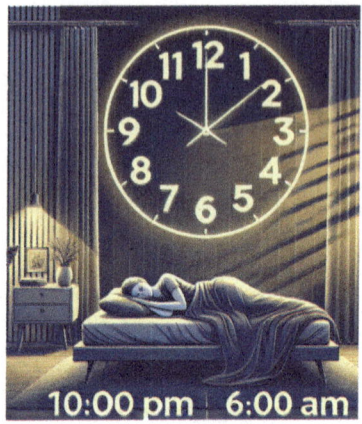

What if I told you that you could fix your posture while you sleep? Crazy, right? But, sleep isn't just about rest; it's an active intervention. Imagine turning 5+ hours of rest into a healing intervention. With the right setup, your body can recover and rest effortlessly—no fancy mattress required. Let's start with one simple tool: *the pillow*.

If you wake up in pain but feel better as the day goes on, could your sleeping position be the culprit? Think about it. You're spending more than 4 hours in one position. That's a lot of time for your body to be in one position, almost as much as an 8-hour work day. If that position isn't supportive, it can create and reinforce dysfunction.

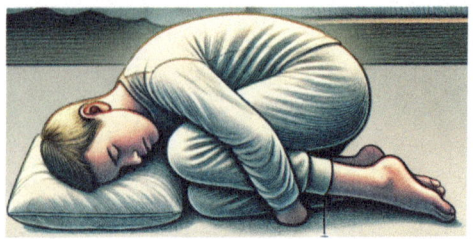

Sure we all toss and turn, but if we don't have the right pillow set up, we might accidentally be spending the equivalent of a 40-hour work week all curled up. If you're constantly changing positions all night, could it be that you're uncomfortable because your body isn't properly supported? Now add on the hours in front of the computer at your full time job. When does your body ever get to actually rest? What if your sleep could heal you? Imagine waking up without stiffness, aches, or pain—just by adjusting your sleeping position.

The good news. You can. Small adjustments in the way you sleep can make the difference.

How do you sleep?

Let's start with some facts:

- 60-70% of people are side sleepers
- 10-20% primarily sleep on their back
- 10% of people sleep on their stomach

Did you know a single pillow can change everything? I know it sounds too good to be true, but after years of working with clients and taking away their pain, this is what we've found. Most people don't realize that one simple pillow adjustment can prevent surgery. I know it sounds "crazy" but I've seen it happen time and time again.

Let's discuss sleeping positions. No, there is no perfect position and no, YOU DON'T NEED A NEW MATTRESS, but there are a few things you should definitely try.

Side Sleeping

Sleeping on your side would be our top choice in sleeping positions—with the proper use of pillows of course. When it comes to our clients that experience lower back pain, hip pain, or knee pain, the biggest game changer is to make sure to sleep with a pillow in between the knees.

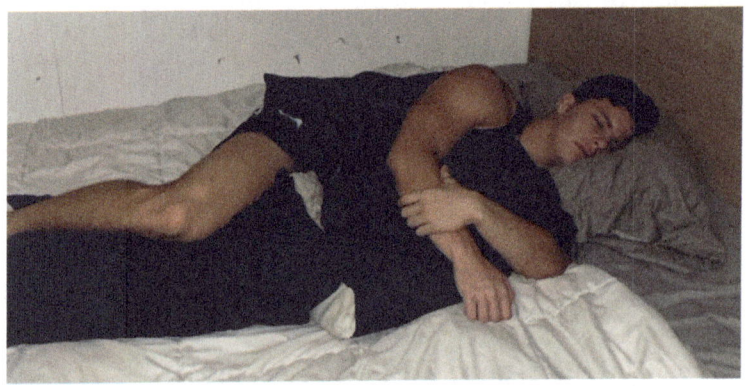

Side sleeping, when done properly, can be your path to pain-free living. Like any choreographed performance, it requires the right props—in this case, four strategically placed pillows that transform a simple sleeping position into a therapeutic intervention. The key to fixing side-sleeping pain isn't a new mattress—it's strategic pillow placement.

The Four Pillow Method: Your Blueprint for Restorative Sleep

How Anna Avoided a Hip Replacement

Anna's story perfectly illustrates the power of proper side sleeping. When she first invited me into her home, she was already scheduled for hip replacement surgery. Months of consultations and X-rays had convinced her of the inevitable. Her hip pain had become unbearable, affecting every aspect of her life. She struggled to get out of bed in the morning and winced every time she climbed the stairs. Sitting too long hurt. Standing too long hurt. Sleep—her only escape—was making it even worse.

During our assessment, I noticed something: Anna was a side sleeper, but didn't have any support between her knees. Each night, her top hip was dropping forward, creating a twisted position that persisted for hours. Imagine standing with your weight shifted entirely to one hip, then staying that way for eight hours straight.

"But I've always slept this way," she protested when I suggested placing a pillow between her knees.

"Let me show you something," I responded. I had her stand and cross one leg over the other, letting her hip drop. "How does that feel after just thirty seconds? Now imagine doing that for eight hours every night."

The realization hit her and we implemented The Four Pillow Method:

- A properly sized pillow under her head to maintain cervical alignment
- A firm pillow between her knees to keep her hips level
- A pillow between her arms, to hug and prevent shoulder strain
- A back pillow to prevent rolling, provide support, and maintain position

Two weeks later, Anna called me, her voice thick with emotion. "I canceled my surgery," she said. "The hip pain... it's almost gone. I can't believe it was my sleeping position all this time!"

The Biomechanical Breakthrough

Each pillow in The Four Pillow Method serves a crucial purpose:

1. Head Pillow: Maintains the natural curve of your neck, preventing cervical strain
2. Knee Pillow: Keeps your hips level and spine aligned, preventing the rotational stress that can trigger everything from sciatica to hip pain
3. Arm Pillow: Supports your upper arm to prevent shoulder compression and rotator cuff strain
4. Back Pillow: Acts as a positional guide, preventing unconscious rolling onto your stomach and allows you to offload your joints, avoiding additional compression from lying on your side

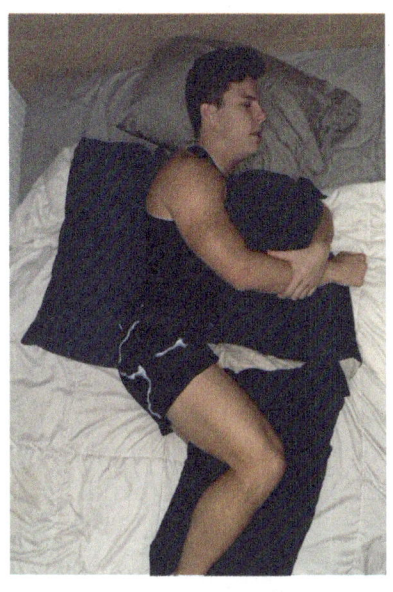

This method isn't just about comfort—it's about creating an environment where your body can truly heal during sleep. This position allows for your joints and muscles to be in a complete resting position. Side sleeping without proper support is like trying to balance a house of cards—eventually, something has to give. The pillow between your knees isn't optional; it's as essential as the foundation of a building. Without it, you're asking your body to maintain an impossible position for hours on end. Your sleeping position is an active intervention. Every night, you're either reinforcing proper alignment or creating new patterns of dysfunction. The choice, and the power to change, lies in how you arrange these four simple pillows.

Any of these pillows can be replaced with a person.

The Knee Pillow Revolution

Every day, I witness the same scene: A client tells me about their chronic pain, their pending surgeries, their lost hope. First thing I ask is about their sleeping position. Almost invariably, there's no pillow between their knees. If you're not putting a pillow between your knees, I can never start to fix your back, hip, or knee pain. And no, it doesn't have to be a fancy and branded "knee pillow"—we actually don't like those. You can use any pillow. At the bare minimum you can even just scrunch up your blankets or use a stuffed animal (I use a squishmallow) so that your hip and pelvic alignment are improved.

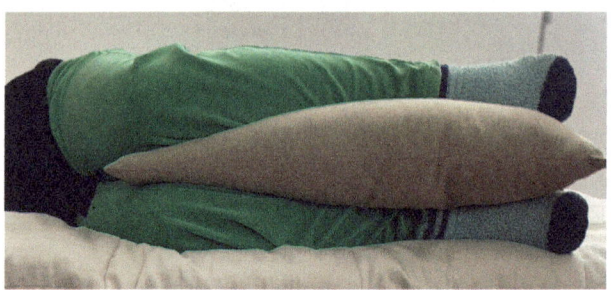

It seems almost too simple. A single pillow, strategically placed, creating cascading effects throughout the body's entire kinetic chain. Yet the results speak for themselves:

- Janet canceled her knee replacement after two weeks of proper side sleeping
- Liz decided not to have a hip replacement due to decrease in symptoms
- Mike's IT band loosened after years of failed treatments
- Lisa's persistent groin pain vanished
- John's chronic low back pain resolved

What fascinates me most are the casual conversations. At parties, in grocery stores, even waiting in line for coffee—when people mention their pain, I share this simple solution. The follow-up messages never cease to amaze me:

"I can't believe it. My back pain is gone."

"I canceled my knee surgery."

"Why didn't any doctor ever tell me this?"

The most powerful part? This isn't a complex medical intervention. It's not expensive therapy or risky surgery. It's just pillows, properly placed, allowing your body to find its natural alignment during the critical hours of sleep.

Every week, someone reaches out after hearing this advice in passing: "That simple thing changed my life." It might sound like an exaggeration, but after years of witnessing these transformations, I understand why. When you spend eight hours every night in proper alignment instead of subtle contortion, your body can finally heal itself. We don't realize how much time we actually spend in bed.

What if I told you the second most important thing you could do is simply hug a pillow? That's right, just a normal pillow. Not a body pillow.

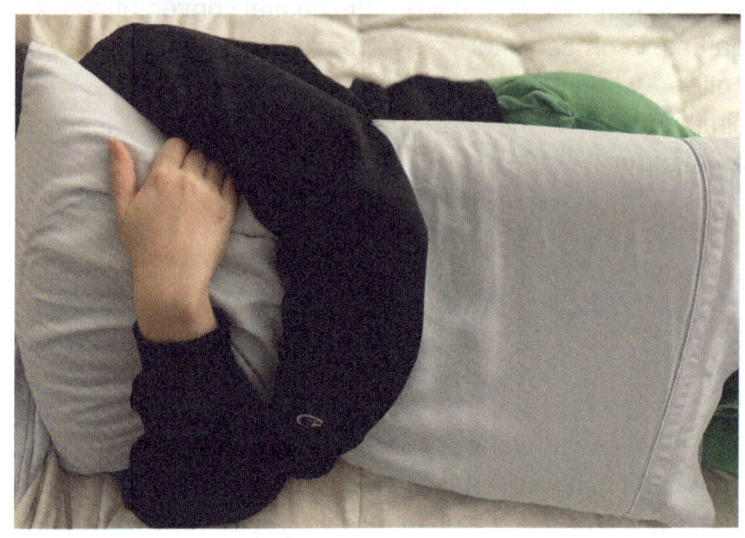

When you hug a regular pillow, it keeps your top shoulder from collapsing forward, which can strain the rotator cuff and compress shoulder structures. This slight elevation and support creates space in the shoulder joint, reducing the risk of impingement. It also helps keep your upper spine and shoulders in better alignment, minimizing stress on the neck and upper back.

A body pillow, on the other hand, is often too large and rigid, which can force your shoulder into an unnatural position or cause you to over-rotate your spine. A simple, soft pillow allows for just the right amount of support without compromising your natural posture.

The Body Pillow Trap: A Hockey Player's Wake-Up Call

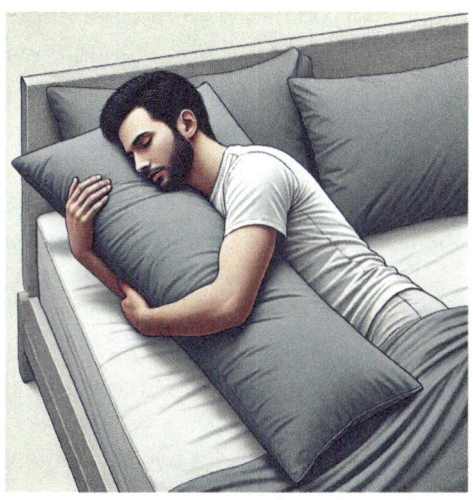

When professional hockey player Marcus invited me into his home, he was battling persistent hip flexor pain that threatened his career. Despite intensive physical therapy, massages, and strength training, the pain lingered, affecting his speed on the ice.

While assessing his bedroom set up, I spotted it immediately: a long, plush body pillow that Marcus proudly declared his "sleep necessity." Like many athletes, he thought more support meant better recovery. But as I watched him demonstrate his sleeping position, I saw the hidden problem unfold.

"Show me how you typically sleep," I asked.

Marcus curled around the body pillow like a koala on a eucalyptus branch, his body forming a tight C-shape. His hips were flexed, his spine curved, his shoulders rounded forward, head resting on pillows that were angled slightly propped on his headboard. What he thought was supporting him was actually locking him into hours of shortened hip flexors and compressed joints.

"Let me show you something," I said. "Stand up and hold that same position you sleep in with the body pillow."

The realization hit him immediately. His athletic body, trained for explosive power and agility, was spending eight hours every night basically doing a sustained crunch.

We replaced the body pillow with two strategically placed separate pillows: one between his knees to maintain hip alignment, and another for his arms to prevent shoulder rounding. The difference was dramatic. This setup offered him the flexibility to adjust his hip angles throughout the night, preventing prolonged stiffness and increasing mobility. By allowing his hips to rest in varied positions, the separate pillows decreased tightness and helped restore natural movement.

A few weeks later, Marcus reported a significant improvement in his hip flexor pain. His morning mobility had improved, and his pre-game warm-ups no longer required extensive hip opening exercises. The change wasn't just about better support—it was about creating freedom for his body to move naturally and recover dynamically through the night, instead of his hip being locked at a certain degree of flexion.

How Stress Shapes Our Sleep

They say stress increases tension, but what we've found is it's often the positions we adopt when we're stressed that create the most problems. When stressed or using a body pillow, you're more likely to curl up in a C like a cashew or candy cane. If that position follows us to bed, it creates hours of unnecessary strain on the spine.

With the head forward all night, the cervical flexor muscles shorten and the extensors lengthen, creating imbalances your body has to combat all day. This makes it harder to maintain an upright posture and hold your head tall. Certain muscles need to stay tight—not stretched—to provide stability and promote extension and neutral alignment.

Try This: Lay against a wall or horizontally against your headboard to check your alignment. Does your head touch the headboard? Notice how far your head is from the wall or headboard. Can you adjust into a neutral position where your head touches? For many, this is a big wake-up call, revealing how forward their head posture has become and how little rest their neck muscles are getting. Try getting your spine more aligned prior to falling asleep. We're not as concerned with how you wake up, awareness is key.

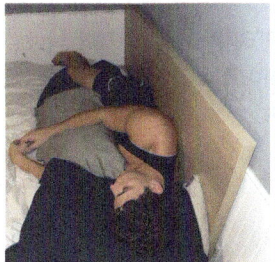 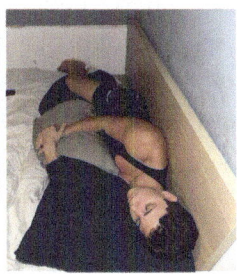

Here's the truth: a 10-minute exercise to reverse your forward head posture can't compete with the 4+ hours of sleeping in neck flexion. Aligning your posture before sleep is essential to reduce strain and allow your body to recover overnight. Give yourself a posture check before you fall asleep.

The Position Prison: Common Sleep Setups That Limit Mobility

1. **The Body Pillow Bind**
   - Locks hips in flexion: shortens hip flexors for > 4 hours per night which is constantly repeated throughout the day with sitting)
   - Forces spine into sustained curve: curls neck and knees to support both into cashew shape)
   - Restricts natural nighttime movement
   - Creates a domino effect of tension through the kinetic chain
2. **Side Sleeping Without Support**
   - Drops top hip forward
   - Twists pelvis
   - Creates compensatory tension in back muscles
   - Forces hip flexors to guard
3. **The Fetal Curl**
   - Shortens entire front of body
   - Restricts diaphragm movement
   - Compresses hip flexors
   - Limits shoulder mobility

The Nightly Shoulder Siege: Beth's Awakening

Beth, a tennis instructor, invited me into her home after months of mysterious shoulder pain. Her serving power had diminished, and she was waking up multiple times each night, tossing and turning, unable to find comfort on her side.

"I used to sleep like a rock," she told me, dark circles under her eyes telling their own story. "Now I can barely make it through two hours without having to shift positions."

When I asked her to show me her typical sleeping position, the problem became immediately clear. Beth was a dedicated side sleeper, but without any support between her arms. Her entire upper body weight was compressing her shoulder into the mattress, creating what we call a "nightly impingement."

"Watch this," I said, having her stand up. "Put your arm in the exact position you sleep in."

She mimicked her side-sleeping pose, arm crushed under her body weight.

"Now hold that position for just two minutes," I instructed.

She couldn't make it past 30 seconds before discomfort set in.

"But I'm doing this for hours every night," she realized, eyes widening.

"Exactly. You're essentially performing a sustained shoulder impingement test on yourself for hours at a time."

The data backed up Beth's experience—many side sleepers struggle with shoulder pain. It's not just bad luck; it's biomechanics.

We ran through some quick tests that confirmed what her sleeping position had created:

- Her impingement test was positive
- The empty can test, which tests for rotator cuff injuries revealed a weakened supraspinatus (a major rotator cuff muscle)
- Her AC joint was tender to the touch

"Here's what's happening," I explained. "Every night, you're creating the perfect storm for shoulder dysfunction":

- Compressed rotator cuff muscles and labrum
- Pinched subacromial space
- Strain to AC joint
- Restricted blood flow to healing tissues

All because of how you're sleeping.

The solution was straightforward: we introduced a pillow between her arms, creating space for her shoulder to rest in a neutral position. For back-sleeping portions of the night, we added a pillow on her chest to prevent her shoulder from rolling forward.

Two weeks later, Beth's transformation was remarkable. "I'm sleeping through the night again," she reported. "My serve is coming back, and that constant ache is finally gone."

The Shoulder Sleep Crisis: A Pattern of Pain

Beth's story is one I see played out in bedrooms across the city. When I arrive for home visits with clients suffering from shoulder pain, the scene is almost always identical: a side sleeper, no pillow between their arms, their shoulder bearing the full weight of their body night after night.

It's one of those moments that makes me want to shout from the rooftops: "Of course you have shoulder pain!" Think about it. When Beth showed me how she slept, her shoulder was essentially being crushed between her body weight and the mattress for 6-8 hours every night.

The pattern is so predictable it's almost maddening:

- Side sleeping without arm support
- Mysterious shoulder pain that won't go away
- Failed physical therapy attempts
- Frustration with "frozen shoulder" diagnosis
- Considering surgical options

All because of one missing pillow.

When I explain this to clients, watching their faces as they make the connection, it's always the same mix of revelation and regret. "You mean I've been doing this to myself?"

Beth's transformation after adding arm support was dramatic but not unique. I see it over and over: proper pillow placement, shoulder pain resolved. It's such a simple fix for what so many consider a complex problem.

Every night that you side sleep without support, you're asking your shoulder to bear a burden it was never designed to handle.

- Upper traps tighten to compensate for the instability
- Thoracic spine gets locked in rotation
- Neck muscles work overtime to maintain head position
- The "free" shoulder actually impinges itself through this forward rolled position
- This is why shoulder pain is rarely just shoulder pain. The compensation patterns ripple through the entire upper body:
    - Neck tension
    - Upper back stiffness
    - Headaches
    - Thoracic mobility restrictions
    - Chronic upper trap tightness

One simple pillow between the arms can prevent this entire cascade of dysfunction. It not only creates space for the bottom shoulder but also maintains proper alignment of the top shoulder, keeping your thoracic spine neutral and your upper traps relaxed.

The Unsung Hero: The Back Pillow Revolution

During Beth's follow-up visit, she revealed something unexpected. Among the four pillows we'd introduced – head, knees, arms, and back – it was the back pillow that had become her secret favorite.

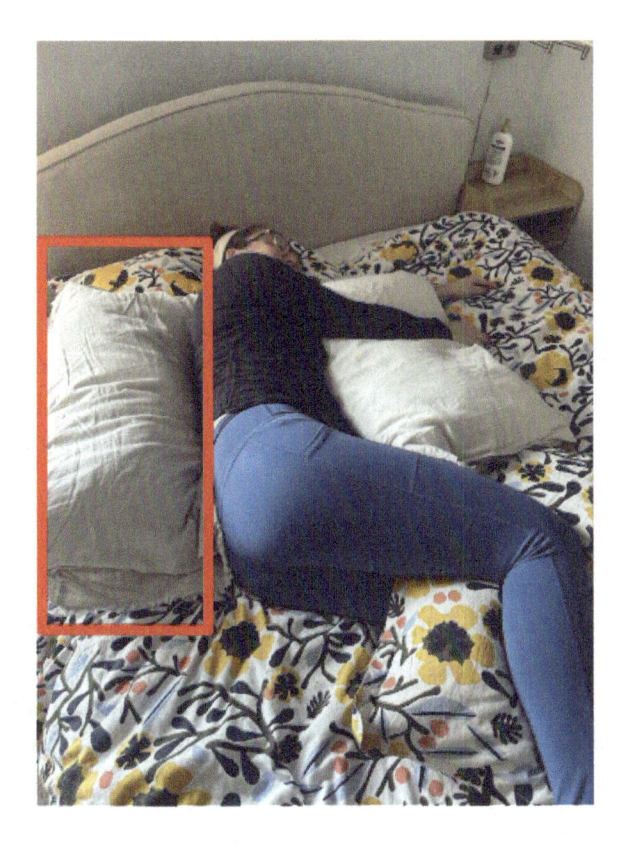

"I never thought the pillow behind my back would matter so much," she confessed. "But it's like having a support system that follows me through the night."

This is a revelation I see time and time again. While clients initially focus on the pillows they can see and feel directly – between the knees and arms – it's often the back pillow that emerges as the unexpected game-changer.

Here's why:

- It creates a gentle support that redistributes weight throughout your body
- When you shift positions during natural sleep movements, you're never "falling" into space
- If you roll to your other side, there's already a pillow waiting to support you
- It prevents compression on your joints from fully weight bearing on one side

I had another client, Gabriel, who was skeptical about the back pillow at first. "I don't roll in my sleep," he insisted. But after one night with the back pillow, he understood. "It's not about preventing rolling," he told me. "It's about feeling supported from all angles. I didn't realize how much tension I was holding until I had that support."

The back pillow is like a loyal friend standing guard while you sleep. It's not just about preventing movement; it's about creating a sense of security that allows your muscles to fully relax. Your body doesn't have to stay vigilant about maintaining position because it knows there's support in every direction.

The Shoulder Sleep Solution

Your shoulder is an incredibly mobile joint, but with that mobility comes responsibility. Every night, you're either supporting its natural alignment, or slowly compromising its function

Think of it this way: Would you stand with all your weight on one shoulder for even five minutes? Of course not. Yet without proper sleep support, that's exactly what you're doing for hours on end.

Back Sleeping

Sleeping on your back is ok if you've got the proper set up. With the "neck taco" technique your head and neck should be cradled inside a fluffy type pillow. At no point should your shoulders or shoulder blades be resting on the pillow. This is what causes the upper trap muscles to be shrugged up and tight all night.

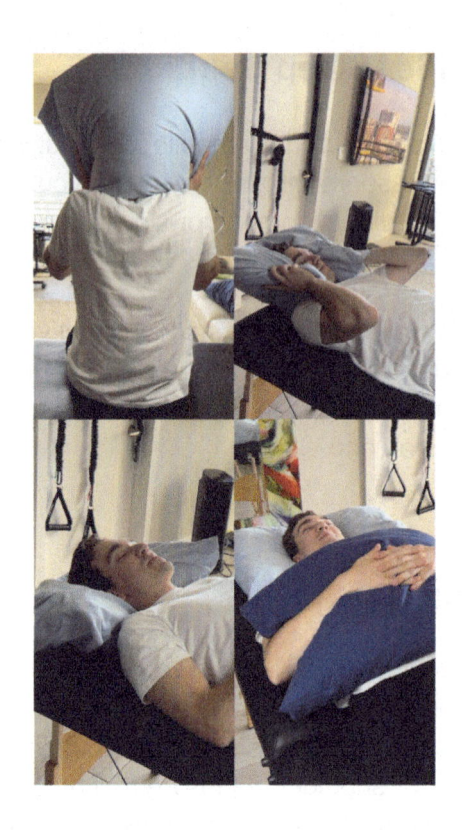

The Neck Taco: A Game-Changer for Back Sleepers

One of my clients, Jake, loved sleeping on his back but often woke up with a stiff neck and headaches. When I asked him to show me how he set up his pillow, the problem became clear: his pillow was flat and wide, sitting under both his neck and shoulders. I introduced him to the "neck taco" technique.

"Sit up," I told him, "and fold your pillow into a supportive curve behind your neck." Once he laid down, the pillow cradled his head from behind and on both sides. Within a week, his stiffness was gone, and he couldn't stop raving about his newfound comfort.

A properly positioned pillow for back sleepers provides support under the neck and head without including the shoulders. The "neck taco" technique ensures your neck stays aligned all night.

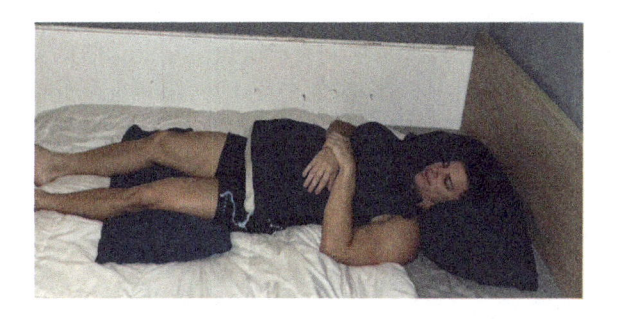

If you sleep on your back with one pillow, you should also sleep with one pillow under your knees—as long as there was no recent surgery or injury. This is known as an antigravity position to offload your spine from the forces of gravity. Think back to the candy cane, the line from the tip of your head to the tip of your toes. If you put too many pillows under your head, you're stressing that line all night. When you put the pillow under your knees, you offload this and give your spine more slack. The problem is that clients often use the incorrect amount of pillows and create extra tension to certain parts of the spine that could lead to the cause of neck or lower back pain.

Have you ever tried sleeping on your back with no pillows? Believe it or not this can be comfortable if you can manage to maintain the chin tucked position. The chin tuck allows for the spine to maintain a neutral position to decrease compression and avoid your neck from hyperextension.

Your deep neck flexor muscles help take the tension off the muscles in the back of your neck that often cause tension headaches. Another important aspect of proper sleeping positions is making sure your pillows are replaced regularly. Allison came to me with a worn-out pillow that had lost its support. She was reluctant to replace it, thinking all pillows were the same. I convinced her to try a firmer, higher-quality pillow, and the results were immediate. "I had no idea how much my old pillow was hurting me," she said. Pillows lose their shape over time. Replace yours regularly to maintain proper support for your neck and spine.

The One-Pillow Rule

- Only one pillow under your head
- Support stops at base of neck
- Shoulders rest flat on mattress
- Regular posture checks before falling asleep

EVERYONE WALKING AROUND HUNCHED OVER IS PUTTING MORE THAN 1 PILLOW UNDER THEIR HEAD

One extra pillow under the head might seem like a good idea when trying to get comfortable, but multiply that one position by 2,920 hours a year, and you're looking at a profound reshape of your body's most fundamental structures. Stacked pillows under the head might seem like a harmless way to be comfortable, but in reality, they're working against your body's natural alignment. Imagine standing up and keeping your neck in the exact position created by two or more pillows under your head—your chin would be almost pointing to the ground.

This forward tilt compresses the cervical vertebrae, strains the neck muscles, and is a significant contributor to the formation of a "neck hump." Sleeping with more than one pillow puts you on the fast track to becoming the candy cane.

Riley's Story: The Misplaced Blame

Riley came to me complaining of chronic neck pain, which he attributed to a car accident five years ago. He was convinced the accident was the sole cause of his discomfort because his MRI showed a herniated disc at C6-C7. "I've never been the same since," he said, convinced his injury was permanent and untreatable.

However, as we dug deeper into his habits, a different picture emerged. Riley was using two pillows under his head every night, certain it was the only way to feel supported. What he didn't realize was that this habit was forcing his neck into an unnatural forward tilt, compressing his cervical vertebrae and significantly contributing to his persistent pain and a visible "neck hump."

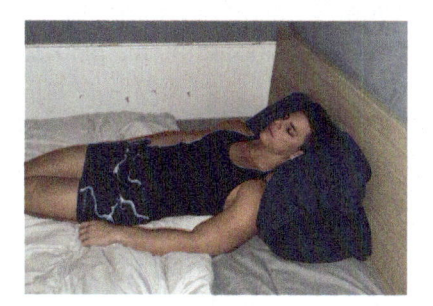

We replaced his two pillows with one thicker, more supportive option tailored to his needs, and the results were transformative.

"My posture has never felt this good," Riley reported after just one month. Not only did his neck pain improve, but his overall posture and energy levels also saw a dramatic shift.

The Headboard Pillow Disaster

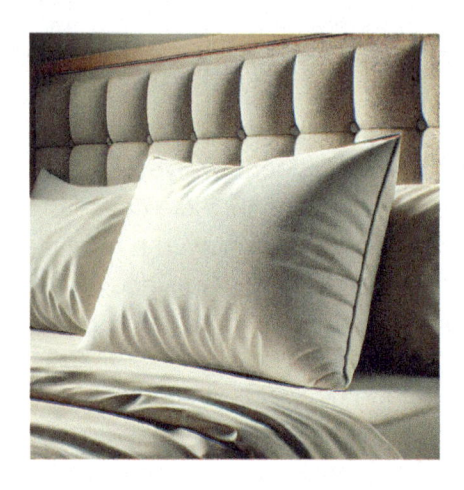

Mark had already undergone one neck surgery and was dreading the thought of another. Despite hours of extensive research and consultations, numerous doctor visits, physical therapy, and ergonomic adjustments, his pain persisted. When I visited his home, the culprit became obvious: he used his headboard as his pillow.

Mark spent every night with his neck angled upward, using the hard headboard as support. This position wreaked havoc on his cervical spine.

Once we replaced the headboard with a proper pillow that supported his neck in a neutral position, his symptoms began to improve. "I can't believe something so simple was causing me so much pain," he said during a follow-up session.

Your pillow's position should support your neck, not push it into unnatural angles. Placing a pillow too close to the headboard creates strain on the cervical spine that builds over hours of sleep.

Hope's Sleep Nightmare

Hope's story was one of silent suffering – severe migraines and TMJ pain that had become her constant, unwelcome companion since recovering from a prolonged illness.

During her extended recovery, Hope had spent countless hours in bed, her body healing, but her movements restricted. What she didn't realize was that her recovery was creating a new form of trauma – one born from seemingly insignificant details that compound over time.

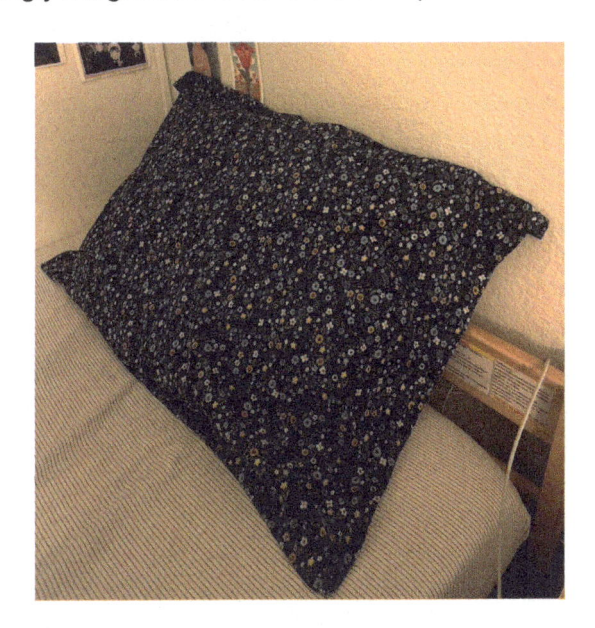

When I visited her home, the source of her pain became apparent. Her bedroom told a story of unintentional self-harm. Her pillow, a misshapen rectangle, was propped awkwardly against the hard headboard, creating an unnatural angle that twisted her neck throughout the night. Each hour of sleep was a subtle assault on her cervical spine, her jaw muscles clenched in a perpetual state of tension.

Look up towards the ceiling, notice your jaw open. The muscles that maintain your jaw in an open position often create headaches and symptoms in the neck. When you look down, your jaw closes, causing clenching at night and sometimes subconscious grinding that fatigue and overwork your muscles all night long.

"Most people don't understand how something as simple as pillow placement can cascade into chronic pain," I explained to her. Her neck was forced slightly upward, creating a microstrain that, over weeks and months, had transformed into the migraines and jaw pain that had become her new normal.

We worked together to reimagine her sleep environment. A supportive pillow that cradled her neck in a neutral position replaced the old setup. It was a minor adjustment – almost undetectable to the untrained eye – but for Hope, it was transformative.

Weeks later, she returned to me, her eyes brighter and her posture more relaxed. The migraines that once controlled her life had dramatically reduced. Her jaw, no longer a constant source of pain, had begun to release its long-held tension.

We've had countless clients swear they only use one pillow and this is why the at home assessment is essential. Many of them accidentally had their pillow partially stacked on another pillow, too close to the headboard creating a tilt, or too close to the edge of the bed causing tension all night to keep the pillow on the bed.

Stomach Sleeping: Breaking the Habit

There's no perfect way to sleep, but if we had to choose, sleeping on your stomach would be the worst position. Most clients we treat that sleep on their stomach claim to be unable to sleep any other way. Chronic neck and lower back pain typically arises from this posture due to excessive compression on your spine from being in spinal extension. Your most "comfortable" position might be your body's greatest enemy.

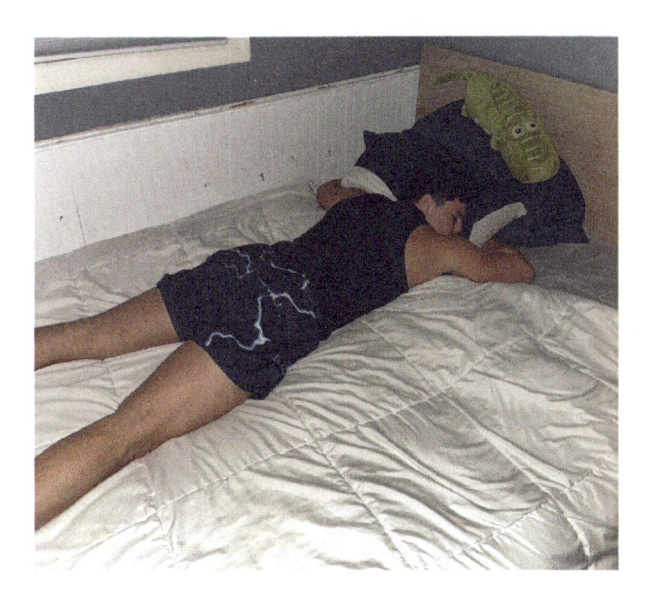

Stomach sleeping doesn't just cause localized pain. It's a full-body assault:

- Neck rotation creates cervical strain
- Lower back hyperextension leads to chronic pain
- Shoulder positioning creates rotator cuff stress
- Increased pressure on internal organs
- Potential nerve compression
- Accelerated spinal degeneration

With our experience, we found that our clients with plantar fasciitis were typically stomach sleepers. While sleeping on your stomach, your ankles are pointed down in a plantarflexed position which shortens your calf muscle and plantar fascia. When you wake up in the morning and stand up, the foot and calf typically feel tight and painful from being in that position all night. We recommend lying with your ankles off the end of the bed if you absolutely have to sleep on your stomach.

Stomach Sleepers & Transitioning Into The Four Pillow Method

The "Four-Pillow Method," isn't just a recommendation—it's a rescue mission for your spine. It helps stomach sleepers transition to side sleeping. Most stomach sleepers I work with are shocked to learn how much damage they're doing. Their neck is rotated 90 degrees, creating constant strain on cervical vertebrae. Their lower back is arched in a way that would make anyone wince. The transition isn't easy. It requires strategy, patience, and what I call "positional retraining."

The Four Pillow Method creates a physical barrier that prevents you from rolling onto your stomach and offloads your joints, gradually retraining your body to find comfort in a side-sleeping position. The Four Pillow Method is made up of:

    1 Head Pillow

    1 Knee Pillow

    1 Arm Pillow

    1 Back Pillow

The Four Pillow Method: Your Blueprint for Restorative Sleep

1. Head Pillow: Your cervical spine's guardian
2. Knee Pillow: Your hip and spine's savior
3. Arm Pillow: Your shoulder's support system
4. Back Pillow: Your positional anchor

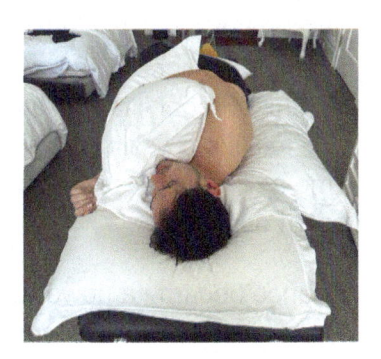

The Hidden Knee Connection to Sleep: A Personal Journey

My own journey with understanding sleep positions began unexpectedly on a soccer field. One moment I was charging for the ball, the next I was on the ground, my patella dislocated. It was a painful lesson that would later transform my approach to treating patients.

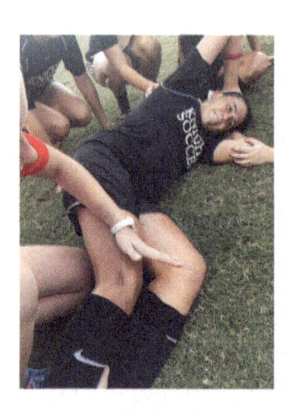

During my recovery, I discovered something crucial: stomach sleeping was impossible. The position created unbearable compression and shear forces on my injured knee. Even after months of rehabilitation, attempting to sleep on my stomach felt like pressing on a bruise. My body was sending me a clear message about the forces this position creates on our joints.

This personal experience became a powerful lens through which I began to see my clients' knee issues differently. Selena, a long-time stomach sleeper, came to me with persistent knee pain and early signs of arthritis. Her nighttime habits weren't just affecting her spine—they were silently aggravating her knee condition.

"But I've always slept this way," she insisted, echoing the same resistance I once felt.

I shared my soccer story with her, explaining how stomach sleeping creates a cascade of pressure through our joints. When you lie on your stomach, your knees bear hours of compression against the mattress. For anyone with cartilage issues, arthritis, or past injuries, this position can be like taking sandpaper to an already sensitive surface.

"Think about it," I told her. "Would you spend eight hours pressing your knee into a hard surface while awake? That's exactly what stomach sleeping does."

The realization hit home. Using the Slight Motion Method's transition techniques, she gradually shifted to side sleeping. Within weeks, her knee pain decreased significantly. "I never made the connection between my sleeping position and my knees," she admitted. "It seems so obvious now."

The Midnight Foot Relief: James's Plantar Fasciitis Story

When I arrived at James's house, he greeted me at the door with a pronounced limp—his morning steps a testament to the agony of plantar fasciitis. Like most sufferers, his first steps each day were excruciating—like walking on broken glass. Multiple physical therapy sessions at clinics had provided temporary relief, but something was missing.

During our assessment, I asked about his sleeping position. "Stomach sleeper, always have been," he declared proudly. "I've tried side sleeping, but I just can't do it. It feels wrong. Unnatural. I've been sleeping on my stomach for forty years."

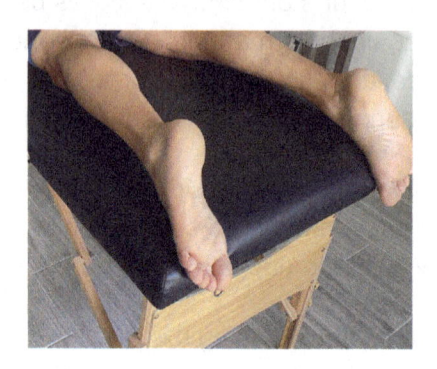

In his bedroom, the evidence of his nightly sabotage became clear. The worn impression on his mattress showed exactly how he slept—prone, with his feet pointed downward. Eight hours of stomach sleeping meant eight hours of pointed toes, his calves and plantar fascia shortened and tightened. Each morning, those first steps weren't just painful—they were his body's protest against the nightly shortening of his posterior chain.

When I explained this connection, James was skeptical but willing to experiment. "But I really can't side sleep," he insisted. "I've tried everything."

That's when I introduced him to what I call the "Neutral Foot Bridge"—a transitional solution for stomach sleepers battling plantar fasciitis. We simply moved his body down the bed so his feet could hang off the edge in a neutral position. No pointed toes. No calf shortening. Just gravity-assisted ankle positioning that maintained length in his posterior chain.

The results were immediate. During our follow-up visit, James reported, "The morning pain was different. Still there, but not as sharp." This small victory opened his mind to the possibility of change.

Over the next few weeks of home visits, we gradually transitioned James to side sleeping using the Slight Motion Method's positioning techniques. The transformation of his morning pain levels were remarkable.

The Plantar Connection

This pattern emerges consistently in my home visits. Nearly every client with plantar fasciitis shares the same story:

- Stomach sleeping
- Pointed toes all night
- Shortened calves
- Morning pain

The solution often lies not in more stretching or orthotics, but in changing this nightly habit. For those resistant to immediate side sleeping, the "Neutral Foot Bridge" serves as a crucial transitional tool.

Your sleeping position isn't just about comfort—it's about maintaining optimal tissue length throughout your body's kinetic chain. Sometimes, the path to healing requires a slight shift in position, a small change that creates ripples of relief throughout your entire system.

The Phone Trap

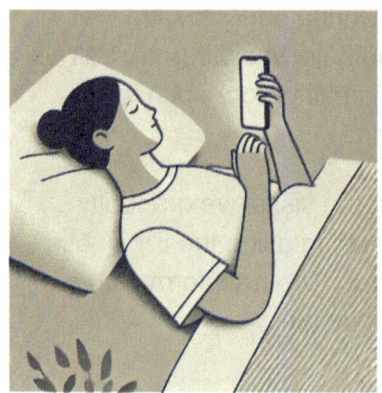

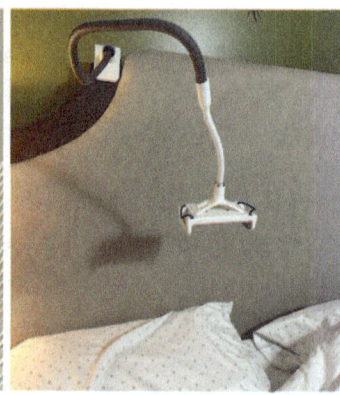

Linda was a busy professional who often scrolled through her phone in bed, lying on her back with the device resting on her chest. When her neck pain worsened, she initially blamed her pillow. During a home visit, I noticed her habit of propping up her phone with her neck craned forward for hours.

I taught her to use a gooseneck phone holder to help prevent her neck from becoming a candy cane at night. This simple device allows you to position your device at eye level, eliminating the need to look down and reduces forward head posture. This upright viewing angle supports a neutral spine position, helping to protect the cervical spine and prevent muscle tension and stiffness.

Investing in a gooseneck phone holder is a small change that can make a big impact. It's a simple upgrade that supports better spinal health while keeping convenience and comfort intact. After implementing this change, Linda's neck pain subsided.

Bonus Wins: Breathing and Mouth Tape

Mouth breathing reduces your body's oxygen efficiency. Nose breathing, on the other hand, allows tiny nasal hairs to filter the air and produces nitric oxide, which dilates blood vessels. This improves blood flow, enabling better oxygenation and recovery during the night, rather than depriving your body of vital support.

Like many clients, Taylor was a chronic mouth breather, waking up groggy and in pain. She started using mouth tape and nose strips, and the difference was night and day. "I'm more rested after four hours now than I used to be after eight," she said.

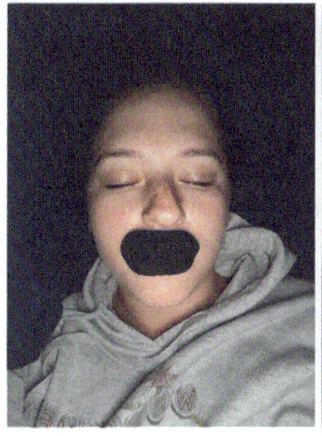

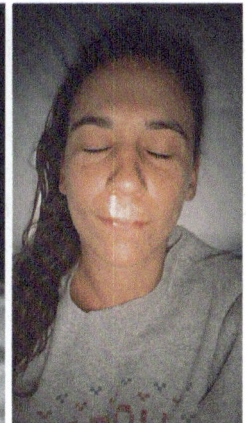

Mouth tape can be a simple way to enhance sleep quality, but consult with your doctor first. My personal life has been changed by mouth taping and nose strips. Many couples report being able to sleep in the same bed for the first time in years since they stopped snoring.

Real Client Breakthroughs

From Recliner to Restful Sleep

One client, who had "tried everything," finally slept in a bed for the first time in over a year after just one session. For months, he had been tossing and turning in a recliner, settling for nonoptimal and restless sleep. Through the Slight Motion Method, we identified habits he didn't even realize were contributing to his discomfort. Now, he's sleeping pain-free, night after night, in a proper bed—and he couldn't be happier.

15 Years of Pain—Gone in One Night

Another client messaged me the day after our session, shocked: "I didn't wake up in pain for the first time in 15 years!" A week later, she wrote, "Day 7—still no pain, scared it will come back." Months later, she continued to send updates like, "Day 90—still no pain!" After years of discomfort, this client finally experienced the relief she thought was out of reach—all thanks to small, intentional changes in her sleep setup.

Goodbye Daily Headaches and Migraines

A client who had suffered from debilitating headaches and migraines every single day found relief after incorporating changes from the Slight Motion Method. By adjusting her sleep posture and eliminating subtle, but harmful misalignments, her headaches stopped entirely for a full month. "I couldn't believe it," she shared. "Going from daily migraines to living almost pain-free has been life-changing." This remarkable transformation shows how optimizing sleep alignment can have ripple effects far beyond the night.

The Slight Motion Revelation

Rest is not inherently healing. Movement is healing. Optimal positioning is healing. Most medical approaches see rest as a passive, neutral state. The Slight Motion Method understands rest as an active intervention—one that requires as much intention and care as any rehabilitation exercise. Extended periods of immobility, especially in nonoptimal positions, can create chronic pain patterns that outlast the original injury.

Your sleep setup is one of the most critical factors in managing pain. If you actually think about it, we spend so much time sleeping! Clients report significant improvements in symptoms by changing their sleep habits and placing pillows in optimal positions. Sleeping is not a passive experience. It's an active intervention you perform every single night. Small changes, like using a single pillow under the head, adjusting its position, or transitioning away from stomach sleeping, can lead to profound improvements.

Remember, sleep isn't just about resting; it's about recovery. By aligning your habits with what your body needs, you can wake up pain-free and ready to conquer the day.

If something as simple as adjusting your pillow can keep you out of surgery, what else are you doing every day that's working against you?

Chapter 3
The Neck Chronicles

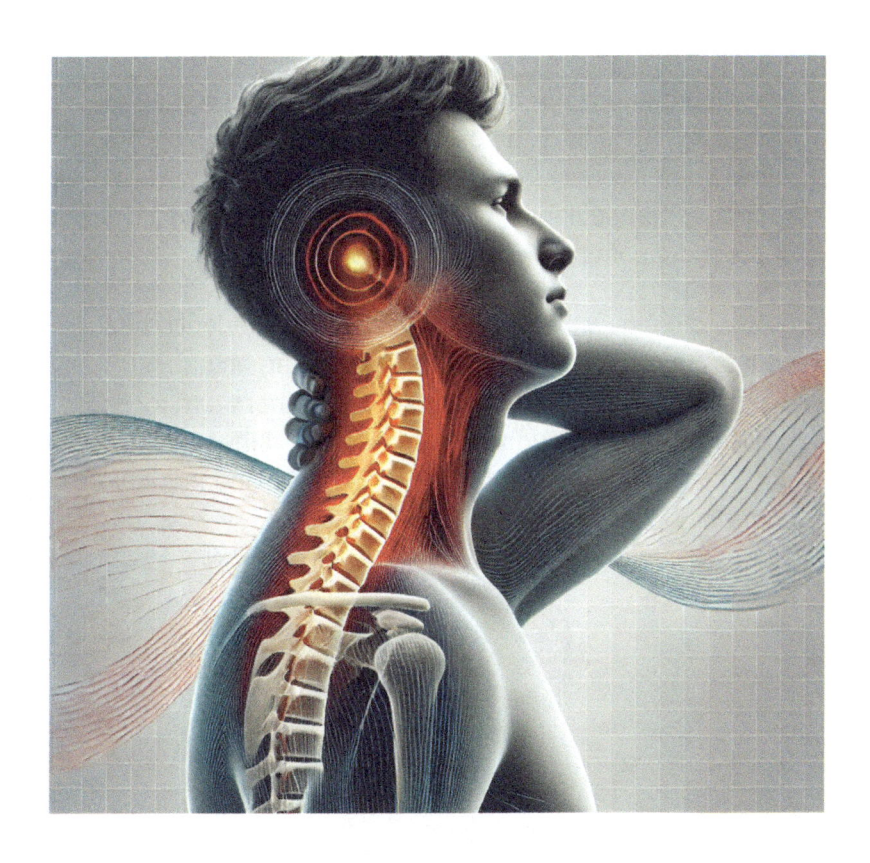

The Neck Chronicles

Why Your Daily Habits Matter More Than You Think

Do you experience neck pain, or do you know someone who does? One time, a young boy jokingly told me, "You know when my neck hurts the most? When you walk by." Humor aside, neck pain is no laughing matter, and it's one of the most common issues I treat.

Research shows that **30-50% of adults** experience neck pain annually[1]; with many reporting it as an actual disability. Many people turn to surgery, others turn to cortisone injections or nerve ablations. But these solutions don't last long because those things ignore the true culprit: your habits.

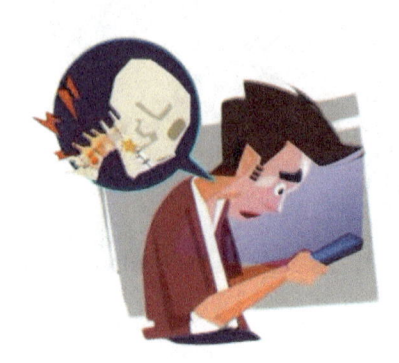

What if small changes in your daily routines– how you hold your phone or set up your work space– could make a difference? One of the biggest factors?
POSTURE—especially while using a phone, tablet, or computer.

Beyond Just "Sit Up Straight"

"Fix Your Posture!"

"Stop Slouching!"

"Sit Up Straight"

How many times have you heard those? But here's what most people don't realize: No one has "perfect posture", but it can always improve. **Your best posture is your next posture** – meaning moving and *slightly* changing positions is far better than trying to stick to an idea of a rigid, "perfect" posture. It's like telling a river to flow perfectly straight; the beauty lies in its natural curves and changes. Making small changes can drastically reduce your neck pain.

"I Love Your Curves"   My Curves:

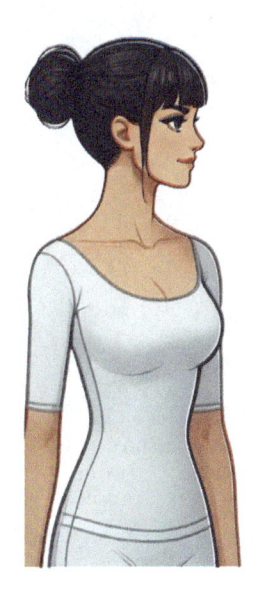

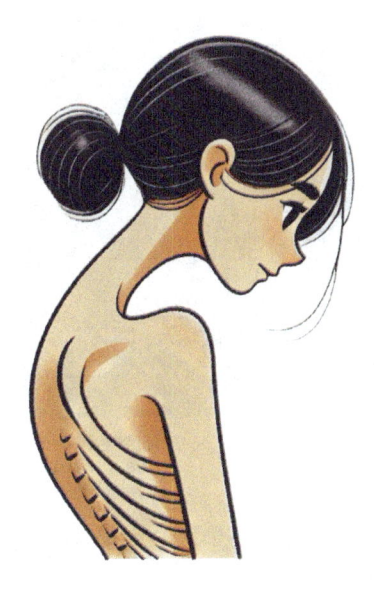

The Modern Neck Crisis

Think of your neck as the bridge between your brain's command center and the rest of your body. Now imagine that bridge handling traffic it was never designed for: hours of looking down at phones, slouching over laptops, and craning at tablets. We're asking our Stone Age spines to adapt to our Space Age habits, and they're crying out in protest.

On average, your skull weighs around 10-12 pounds. For every 15 degrees your head tilts forward, you add an additional 10 pounds of stress to your neck, shoulders, back, and spine. Now imagine that strain compounded hour after hour, as you scroll or type. 40 pounds would be equal to carrying a 4 year old on your shoulders.

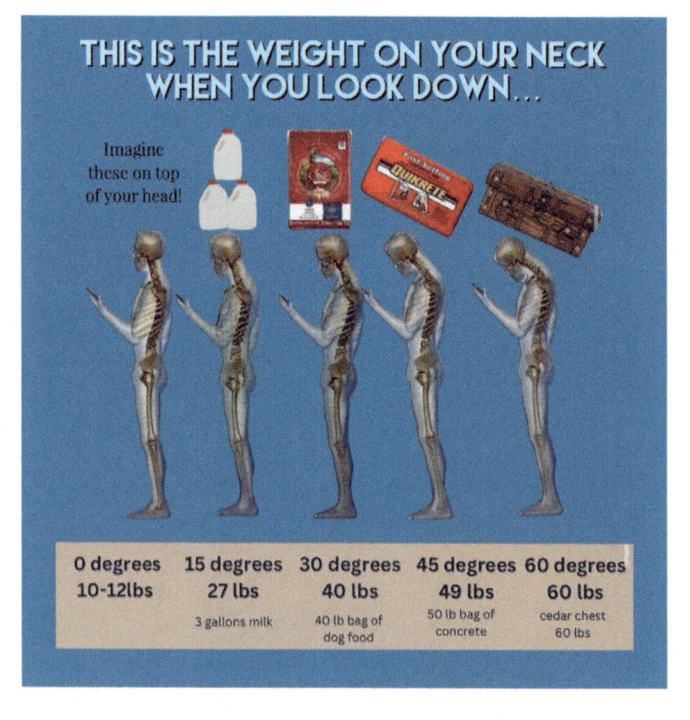

THIS IS THE WEIGHT ON YOUR NECK WHEN YOU LOOK DOWN...

Imagine these on top of your head!

0 degrees	15 degrees	30 degrees	45 degrees	60 degrees
10-12lbs	27 lbs	40 lbs	49 lbs	60 lbs
	3 gallons milk	40 lb bag of dog food	50 lb bag of concrete	cedar chest 60 lbs

This chronic forward head posture, often called "text neck," not only strains your neck muscles, but also disrupts the Superficial Back Line (SBL)—one of the key myofascial lines identified by Tom Myers, author of Anatomy Trains: Myofascial Meridians[2]. The SBL extends from the soles of your feet, through the calves, hamstrings, and spine, to the top of the skull. When your head tilts forward, the tension runs through this entire line, pulling on the hamstrings, spine, and lower back. This is why tight hamstrings or lower back pain often accompany neck pain—everything is connected along these fascial lines.

The Reality Check

Here's something to consider: Your neck moves about 600 times per hour during waking hours. These movements are either reinforcing good patterns or contributing to dysfunction.
By the end of this chapter, you'll understand:

- Which of your daily habits are secretly sabotaging your neck health
- How to modify these habits without turning your life upside down
- Why traditional treatments often fail to provide lasting relief
- Practical strategies you can implement immediately

Remember: Your neck's health isn't determined by one big decision but by hundreds of small choices you make every day. Let's explore how to make those choices count.

The Laptop Lie: Why Your Computer's Name Is Deceiving You

Where do you usually use your phone, tablet, or Kindle? Are they sitting on your lap or too low on a table? This might seem harmless, but holding your devices, especially these heavier ones incorrectly can create serious strain on your neck, shoulders, and wrists.

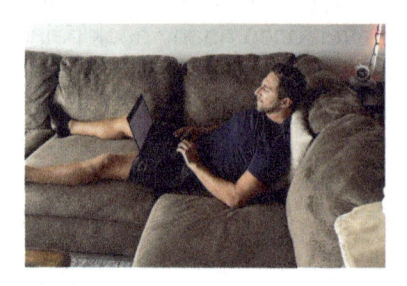

"But it's called a laptop," Alex said with a frustrated laugh. Alex is a successful software developer in his early thirties, who came to us with persistent neck pain, tight hamstrings, and what he described as a growing "hump" at the base of his neck. Despite regular stretching and massage therapy, nothing seemed to help.

When I visited his home office, I found him working exactly as he had for the past five years: curled over his laptop like a question mark, his spine curved into what I call the "gremlin position."

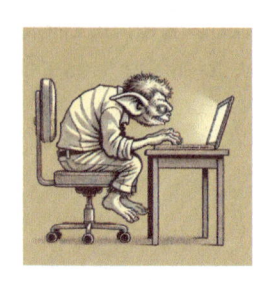

"I've tried everything," he explained, demonstrating his daily stretching routine. "I spend twenty minutes every morning working on my hamstrings, but they're still tight. I get massages twice a month for my neck, but the pain always comes back."

What Alex didn't realize was that his body was telling a story:

- Neck curved forward to see the screen
- Spine compressed in the shape of a candy cane
- Nervous system pulled tight like a string
- Hamstrings responding to the overall tension

"Imagine your body is like a puppet with strings", I said. "When you pull one string - like your neck forward - everything else has to compensate. Your tight hamstrings aren't the problem; they're a symptom of your spine being pulled out of position all day." We can never fix your tight hamstrings if you're working on a laptop with no laptop stand.

His eyes widened as I explained how his laptop position was affecting his entire body. Then he asked, "But what am I supposed to do? I need to work."

The solution was simpler than he expected: a proper laptop stand that brought his screen to eye level, plus an external keyboard and mouse. A laptop stand is non negotiable. I can never fix anything about you if you don't use one.

"This goes everywhere with you," I emphasized. "To coffee shops, to the airport, everywhere. Your laptop stand is now as essential as your phone charger."

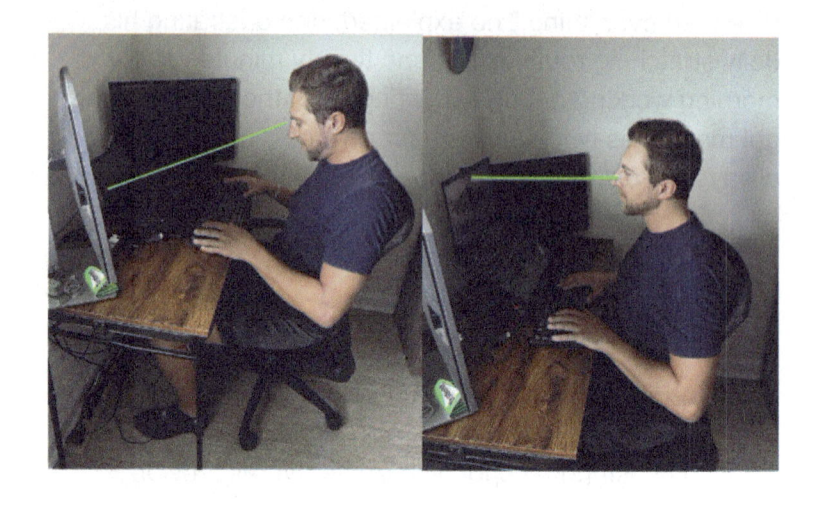

"But that seems so... inconvenient," he protested.

"More inconvenient than chronic pain?" I asked.

Two weeks later, Alex called me. "I can't believe it," he said. "My hamstrings feel looser even though I've stopped stretching them so much. And my neck... the pain is almost gone."

Your body is an interconnected system. Like a chain, tension in one area affects everything else. You can stretch your hamstrings all day, but if your spine is constantly pulled out of position, that tension will keep returning.

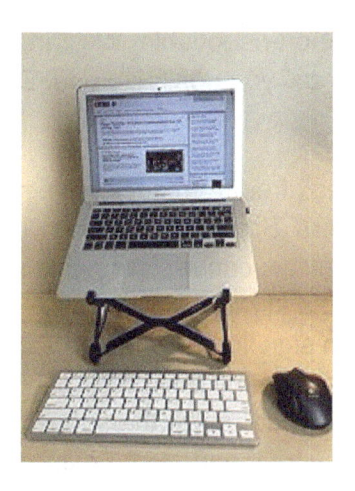

Take a "posture audit" of your day:

- Where is your screen in relation to your eyes?
- Is your spine curved or straight?
- Are you creating a chain reaction of tension?
- What "convenient" positions might be causing problems?

A few days later, Alex sent me a photo of his mobile work setup - laptop stand, external keyboard, and mouse - arranged perfectly at a coffee shop. "I used to think I looked silly setting all this up," his message read. "Now I realize I looked much sillier, hunched over like a gremlin. And the best part? No more pain."

Now when clients come to me with neck pain and tight hamstrings, one of my first questions is "What does your office setup look like?" You'd be surprised how many people think a standup desk is the answer. Most of the time it's not about standing up, it's about not looking down.

A laptop stand is non-negotiable. We can never fix anything about you if you don't use one. Don't be the candy cane.

If you want to break free from neck pain, how you hold your device matters. Small adjustments, like using a stand to elevate your device, can restore healthy alignment across your spine and reduce strain along your fascial lines. We've seen significant improvements in clients who make these changes early on in their pain cycle. The sooner you adjust your habits, the sooner you'll stop the cycle of repetitive strain and start moving toward lasting relief. Simple equipment that elevates the device to eye level, like a gooseneck stand or device holder, can drastically reduce tension on the neck and upper body. If you're using your devices for more than 10 minutes a day, proper ergonomics are non-negotiable.

The Visible Solution: Why Out of Sight Isn't Always Right

The sleek startup office looked like a magazine spread - open floor plan, standing desks, and what seemed like every ergonomic gadget available. But something wasn't working. Despite my previous visit and recommendations, team members were still experiencing neck and back pain.

Heather, the Head of Operations, greeted me with a knowing smile. "We need to show you something," she said, leading me to a storage closet. There, stacked neatly on shelves, were all the collapsible laptop stands I'd recommended months ago.

"They're beautiful, aren't they?" she said with a touch of irony. "Too beautiful, actually. Our founders would fold them up after each use, tuck them away, and completely forget about them. They're in 'grind mode' - they sit down, open their laptops, and dive straight in."

That's when everything clicked. The very feature I thought would be an advantage - portability - had become a liability. The stands were so easy to put away that they were never there when needed.

Sometimes the best solution isn't the most convenient one:

- Portable doesn't always mean practical
- Visibility drives behavior
- Friction can be functional
- Permanent reminders beat perfect design

The solution? We replaced the sleek, collapsible stands with bulky, decidedly less adjustable ones. They weren't pretty. They couldn't be tucked away. They were, as one founder put it, "impossible to ignore."

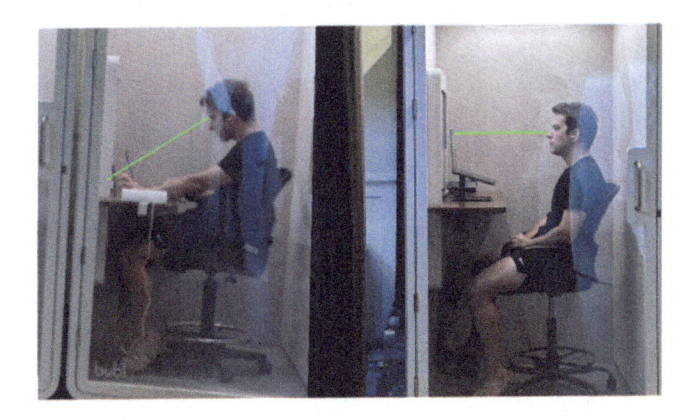

At the next visit, Heather reported a surprising change. "Nobody loves how these stands look," she laughed, "but everyone's using them. The funny thing is, the team is starting to notice other benefits too: less neck pain, better focus, even improved energy levels."

Make your ergonomic tools impossible to ignore:

- Keep stands permanently on desks
- Make proper positioning the default
- Create visual reminders of good posture
- Use equipment that demands attention

As one founder told me later, "I used to think good posture was about willpower. Now I realize it's about making it harder to sit wrong than to sit right."

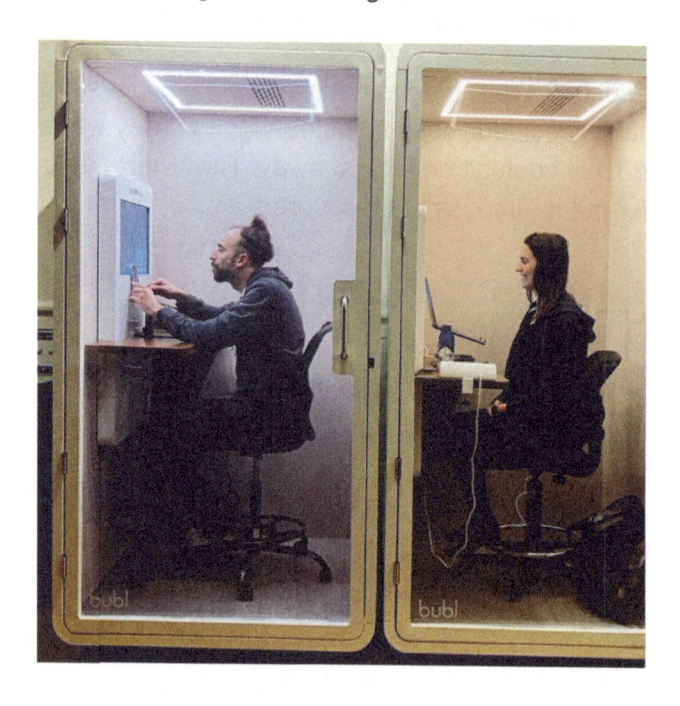

The Side-Glance Syndrome: A Story of Monitor Misalignment

I'll never forget walking into Michael's home office. He was a successful engineer who had been dealing with debilitating neck pain for months. He spent thousands on chiropractic treatments and outpatient physical therapy without lasting relief. As he showed me his workspace, I noticed something right away - his dual monitors were arranged in an L-shape, forcing him to constantly turn his head to the left.

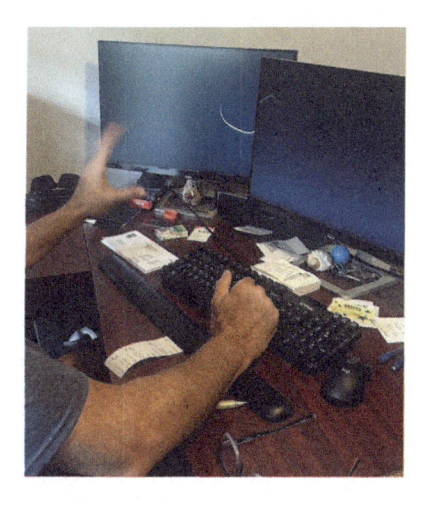

"But I've had this setup for years," he protested when I pointed it out. "And the pain only started recently."

"How many hours are you working now compared to before?"
I asked.

His face changed as he made the connection. "Well, since we went remote... probably double."

Think about it:

- 30-degree head turn
- 8-10 hours daily
- Hundreds of neck rotations
- Sustained muscle tension on one side = Recipe for chronic pain

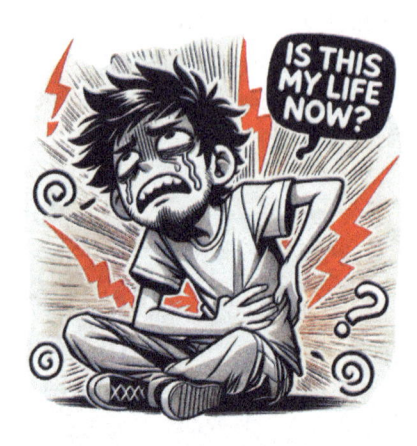

Constantly turning your head to one side to view a monitor might seem like a minor position shift, but over hours, days, and months, it leads to significant muscle imbalance. As your head repeatedly tilts and turns in one direction, the muscles on one side of the neck are lengthened, while those on the other side are shortened. This imbalance can lead to tension headaches, nerve compression, and reduced flexibility. By centering the primary monitor and aligning it slightly above eye level, we encourage symmetrical posture, distributing the strain evenly across both sides of the neck and shoulders, which helps prevent pain and fatigue.

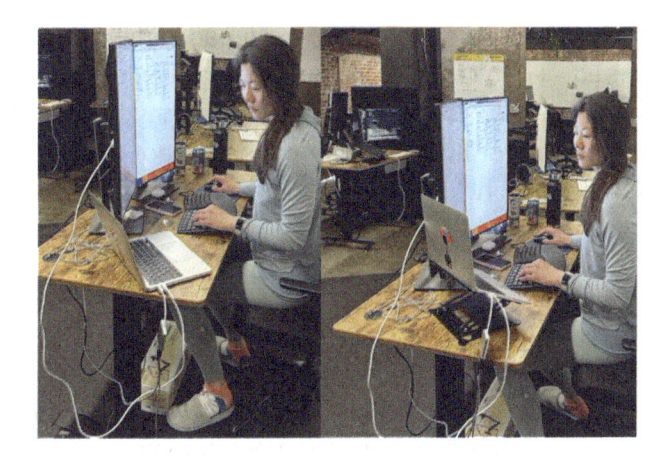

For Michael, we made three simple changes:

1. Centered his primary monitor directly in front
2. Positioned it slightly above eye level (not at eye level as traditionally recommended)
3. Created a rotation schedule for his second monitor

"But what about ergonomic guidelines?" he asked. "Everyone says monitors should be at exact eye level."

"Here's the problem with that," I explained. "Eye level changes based on how you're sitting. When you set your monitor at exact eye level, you often end up slouching to match it. By placing it slightly higher, we encourage your core to engage and your spine to lengthen naturally."

We also established a simple protocol:

- Switch second monitor side every few days
- Adjust monitor heights by 1-2 degrees every 30 minutes
- Stand up during transitions
- Engage core before adjusting posture

Two weeks later, Michael's neck pain had significantly decreased. "I can't believe something so simple made such a difference," he told me. "And the funny thing is, I'm actually more productive now because I'm not constantly fighting discomfort."

Ask yourself:

- Is your monitor directly in front of you?
- Do you have to turn your head to see any screen?
- Is your monitor height encouraging good posture?
- How often do you change your setup?

This could be YOU!

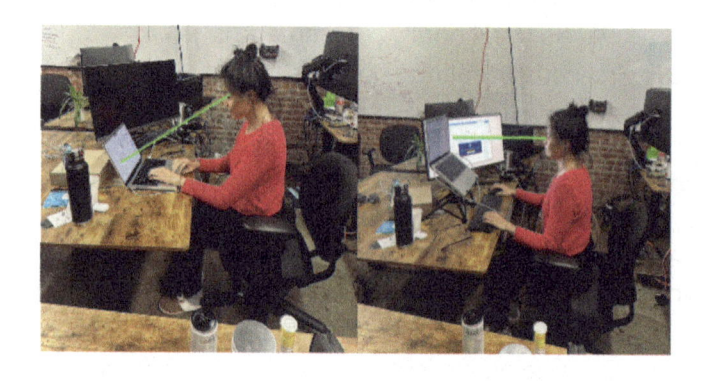

Monitor positioning affects more than just your neck:

- It influences entire posterior fascial chain,
- Impacts core engagement,
- Affects shoulder blade positioning, and
- Can even influence lower back posture

A week later, Michael had implemented these principles with his team. "We now have a 'monitor movement protocol,'" he laughed. "Everyone thought I was crazy at first, but now they're all doing it."

The best monitor position isn't static - it's dynamic. Your body needs different angles and positions throughout the day.

As we know: "The best posture is your next posture."

The Subtle Head Tilt That Almost Led to Surgery

Amy was at her breaking point when she first came to see me. A successful customer service manager, she was experiencing severe neck pain and nerve symptoms that shot down her right arm into her fingers. Three different surgeons had suggested surgical intervention for what they suspected was a herniated disc.

"I've tried everything," she explained, unconsciously rubbing her right hand. "Physical therapy, injections, even changed my entire workstation setup. Nothing helps." Her voice cracked slightly. "Surgery feels like my only option left."

But something about her story nagged at me. The pain had started gradually about six months after transitioning to remote work, and it was always worse after her workday. During our conversation, I noticed a subtle but consistent pattern - she slightly tilted her head during our entire discussion.

"Tell me about your cochlear implant," I said, gesturing to her left ear.

Her eyes widened. "What does that have to do with my neck?"

"Humor me," I replied. "Walk me through a typical work call."

She demonstrated her usual position at her desk, and there it was - that same subtle tilt, barely noticeable unless you were looking for it. Her speakers were positioned on her right side, and she unconsciously tilted her head just a few degrees to better capture the sound.

Think about what this meant:

- Slight head tilt of perhaps 5 degrees
- Maintained for 5-6 hours per day of calls
- Muscles working constantly to hold position
- Nerves compressed in the same pattern
- All happening without awareness

"But it's such a tiny movement," she protested when I explained. "Could that really cause this much pain?"

Consider this:

A 5-degree tilt + Held for 300 minutes daily
    X 5 days a week X 52 weeks a year
        = Thousands of hours of subtle strain
        = **PAIN**!

The solution was surprisingly simple:

- Repositioned her speakers directly in front of her
- Adjusted her microphone settings for better pickup
- Created awareness of her unconscious tilt

Two weeks later, Amy called me, emotion in her voice. "I canceled my surgical consultation," she said. "The pain... it's almost gone. I can't believe I was about to have surgery for something so simple."

Sometimes the most damaging movements aren't the dramatic ones - they're the subtle compensations we make without realizing it. Our bodies are remarkably adaptable, but even small adjustments, when maintained for hours, can create significant problems.

Take a "compensation audit" of your day:

- Are you tilting your head during calls?
- Do you lean toward sound sources?
- Have you adapted your posture for any devices?
- What subtle movements have become habits?

A few weeks later, Amy had become almost evangelical about subtle positioning. "I notice these tiny adjustments everywhere now," she told me. "It's amazing how something so small can make such a big difference."

In this case, the head tilt created constant, one-sided tension in her neck muscles, leading to nerve compression that affected her arm. When muscles on one side of the neck are engaged in this way, they compress nearby nerves and restrict blood flow, potentially causing numbness or tingling.

Adjusting her speakers to face her directly reduced the need for head tilt, allowing her muscles to relax evenly on both sides, alleviating the unnecessary strain on nerves and blood vessels.

The Two-Finger Typist: A Story of Hidden Neck Strain

Lisa was proud of her ergonomic workspace. "I've got everything perfectly positioned," she told me during our first meeting. "Standing desk, ergonomic chair, monitor at the right height - I've checked all the boxes." Yet despite her careful setup, her neck pain persisted.

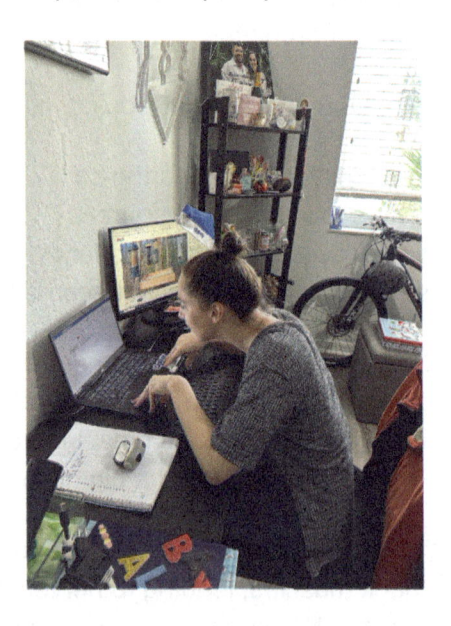

We investigated her work station and noticed while her monitor was perfectly positioned, she kept looking down every few seconds as she typed.

Each glance was brief - just a fraction of a second - but they added up to hundreds of downward head tilts every hour.

"Can you type 'Slight Motion PT' for me?" I asked. "Without looking down?"

She hesitated, fingers hovering over the keyboard. "I... actually need to look," she admitted, ducking her head to find the keys. "I never learned proper typing. I'm a two-finger typist - always have been."

Let's break down what this meant:

> 2-3 downward glances per sentence + about 30 degrees of neck flexion each time
>
> = Hundreds of glances per hour
>
> = Thousands of neck movements per day

"But they're just quick looks," she protested when I explained the impact. "It's not like I'm holding my head down."

Think of your neck like a door hinge:

- Each movement creates micro-wear
- Frequency matters as much as duration
- Repeated patterns create lasting tension
- Small movements accumulate big effects

We calculated that on an average workday, Lisa was looking down at her keyboard over 2,000 times.

That's 2,000 times her neck muscles had to engage to lower and raise her head. Do you ever do 2,000 reps of an exercise at the gym?

The solution wasn't what she expected:

- Online typing course (15 minutes daily)
- Temporary sticky notes on keys for reference
- Timer to practice touch-typing in short bursts
- Gradual reduction of keyboard glances

"Learning to type properly at my age?" she laughed skeptically. "Isn't that like learning a new language?"

A few weeks later Lisa's investment was already paying off. "My typing is still slow," she admitted, "but my neck feels so much better. I never realized how much those little looks down were costing me."

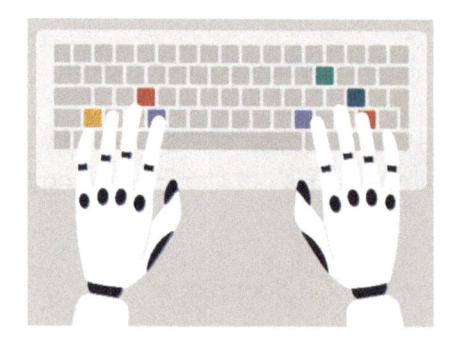

Try this quick typing test:

- Can you type your name without looking?
- What about your email address?
- Could you write a full sentence eyes-forward?
- How often do you catch yourself looking down?

Sometimes the path to pain relief isn't about changing our equipment, it's about changing our skills. As Lisa discovered, investing in basic typing proficiency wasn't just about productivity; it was an investment in her physical health as well.

Set a timer for 2 minutes and try to type without looking down. Notice:

- When do you automatically look down?
- Which keys cause the most uncertainty?
- How does your neck feel staying in position?
- What percentage of time can you maintain forward gaze?

Before our next PT session, Lisa had become a touch-typing evangelist. "People think I'm crazy when I tell them learning to type properly fixed my neck pain," she told me. "But it's true. Sometimes the smallest changes make the biggest difference."

Each time we look down at a keyboard, even for a brief moment, the neck bends and the muscles re-engage. Over thousands of glances downward, this repetition leads to muscle strain and joint wear. The cumulative effect resembles "text neck," where frequent neck flexion leads to postural misalignment and chronic pain. By improving typing proficiency, Lisa reduces her need to look down, allowing her neck to stay aligned with her spine. This adjustment minimizes repetitive strain, leading to fewer instances of neck flexion and creating a healthier baseline posture. The best ergonomic setup in the world can't compensate for thousands of daily neck movements.

Sometimes the solution isn't in our equipment, it's in our skills. If that's not realistic, consider using speak to text more often.

When "Taking It Easy" Takes Its Toll

Tom's story started with a simple flu that knocked him flat for two weeks. But what began as a temporary illness spiraled into months of debilitating neck pain, radiating arm symptoms and pain and numbness into the fingers. By the time he came to me, he was caught in what he called a "recovery paradox" - the more he tried to rest and recover, the worse he felt.

"I'm doing everything right," he insisted, his voice tinged with frustration. "I'm taking it easy, staying off my feet, giving my body time to heal."

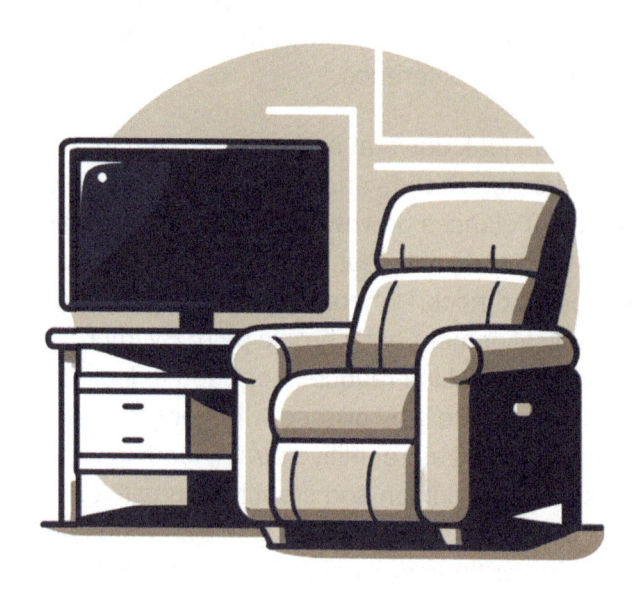

When I visited his home, I found him in what he'd designated his "recovery chair" - a plush recliner that seemed perfectly comfortable. But something caught my eye: the chair was positioned to the left of his television, forcing him to rotate his head to the right to watch.

"How many hours do you spend here?" I asked.

"Most of the day now," he admitted. "I used to be active, but with this pain... Netflix has become my best friend." He demonstrated his typical position, and there it was - his neck turned approximately 30 degrees to the right, held in that position for hours.

What Tom didn't realize:

- "Rest" doesn't mean static positioning
- Recovery requires proper alignment
- Comfort doesn't always equal healing
- Static positions can create new problems

"But I need to rest and recover," he protested when I explained how his TV setup was actually preventing healing. "Where else am I supposed to sit?"

Consider this:

30 degree neck rotation + 6-8 hours of TV daily

= Muscles held in constant tension & Nerves compressed in one position

= **Recipe for chronic pain**

We made two simple changes:

1. Repositioned his chair directly in front of the TV
2. Adjusted TV height for his reclined viewing position

One week later, Tom called me. "I can't believe something so simple made such a difference," he said. "The pain started improving almost immediately."

Recovery isn't just about rest - it's about smart rest. As I explained to Tom, "Your body needs to heal, but it needs to heal in the right position."

Take a "recovery position audit":

- Where is your screen in relation to your seating?
- How long do you maintain one position?
- Does "comfortable" mean "good for you"?
- Are your rest positions actually restful?

Tom had transformed his approach to recovery. "I used to think healing meant staying still," he told me. "Now I understand it's about moving right, not moving less."

This experience changed how I approach recovery protocols. Now when clients tell me they're "taking it easy," I always ask:

- Easy on what?
- Easy in what position?
- Easy for how long?

Tom's story reminds us that sometimes our efforts to heal can actually hinder recovery. As he learned, the path to feeling better isn't always about doing less - it's about doing things right.

While rest is important, prolonged periods in any one position can cause issues. In Tom's case, his constant neck rotation while watching TV was putting one-sided strain on his neck, which interfered with his healing. By moving his chair directly in front of the TV, and elevating his TV, Tom was able to watch comfortably without needing to rotate his neck, which allowed his muscles to relax evenly and encouraged a more balanced healing process.

The Professor's Pain: A Story of Literary Love and Neck Strain

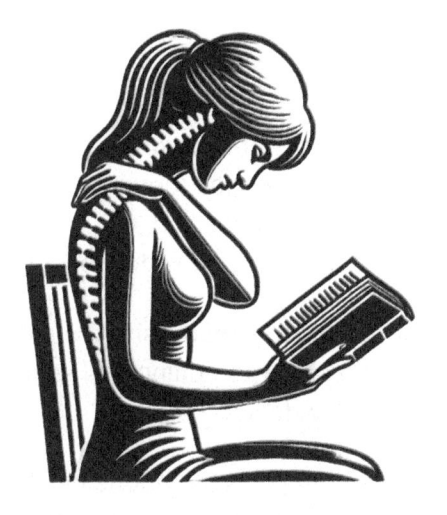

Diana, a literature professor, came to me with what she called her "occupational hazard" - chronic neck pain that had become so severe she dreaded the reading she once loved. "Books are my life," she explained, unconsciously rubbing her neck. "But lately, every page feels like it's costing me physically."

During our first session, I asked her to show me how she typically reads. She pulled out a thick novel from her bag and immediately assumed what I've come to call "The Scholar's Slump" - chin tucked, neck flexed, book resting in her lap. The position was so natural to her, she didn't even realize she was doing it.

"How many hours do you read like this?" I asked.

"Well, I have to review student papers, prepare lectures, keep up with new publications..." She thought for a moment. "Probably four or five hours a day. More during grading periods."

Think about the physics:

- 10-15 pounds of head weight
- Neck flexed 45 degrees forward
- Hours of sustained position
- Multiplied across every reading session

"But this is how I've always read," she protested when I explained the strain she was putting on her neck. "How else am I supposed to do it?"

I asked her to bring her book to various locations - her office, favorite coffee shop, even the campus quad - to show me her typical reading positions. Each setting revealed the same pattern: head down, neck flexed, hours of static positioning.

"Watch this," I said, taking her book and holding it higher. "Notice how your spine naturally straightens when the book rises to eye level."

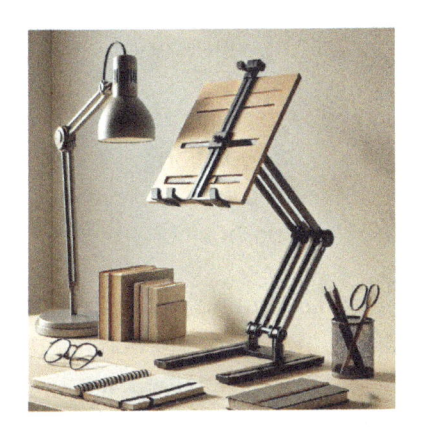

We created location-specific solutions:

- Office: Adjustable book stand on desk
- Home: In a rocking chair NOT on a couch, holding book or iPad up
    - Gooseneck stand
- Travel: Portable stands for airplanes and cafes

A few weeks later, Diana called me, excitement in her voice. "I just finished grading sixty papers," she said, "and my neck doesn't hurt. This is revolutionary."

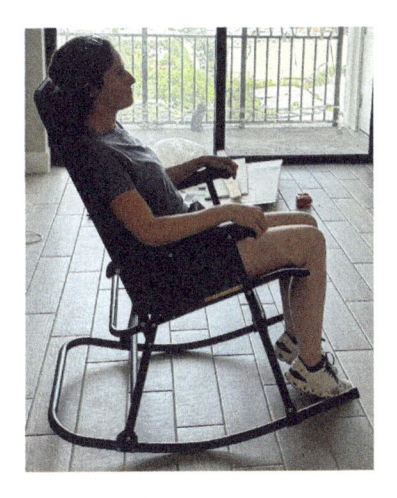

Take a "reading audit" of your day:

- Where do you typically read?
- How long in each position?
- What surfaces or props are available?
- Could the book be positioned higher?

The next semester, Diana had become an advocate for ergonomic reading. "I've started teaching my students about this," she told me. "They think it's amusing that our first literature lesson is about how to hold their books, but their necks will thank me later."

Sometimes the most damaging positions are the ones we've done for so long we don't even question them. As Diana discovered, loving books doesn't have to mean sacrificing your neck. The joy of reading shouldn't come with physical pain. Sometimes the smallest adjustments - like raising your reading material - can make the biggest difference in how you feel.

Holding a book in one's lap while reading causes a forward head posture, which places strain on the neck and upper back. The "scholar's slump," exerts pressure on the muscles and joints over time, contributing to pain and tension. By elevating her book to eye level, Diana no longer needs to crane her neck forward. This small change keeps her head, neck, and spine in a neutral position, distributing the weight of her head more evenly and reducing strain on her neck.

The Hidden Cost of Looking Down: Could Your Phone Lead to Surgery?

What if the way you hold your phone today could determine whether you'll need surgery tomorrow? It's not an exaggeration. Every time you tilt your head down to check your device, you're putting enormous strain on your neck and spine.

The Numbers Don't Lie:

- **At chest level:** Your head exerts up to **60 pounds** of pressure on your spine—equivalent to the weight of a small child!
- **Looking down and to the side:** That's even worse, combining forward tilt with rotation for maximum strain.

But it's not just about your neck, your entire body feels the impact. Every time you look down, you contribute to the "candy cane position," where your spine curves unnaturally under strain. This isn't just a neck issue; it's a whole-body problem. A curved spine creates tension that ripples through your shoulders, lower back, hamstrings, and even your wrists. That's why habits like slouching over your phone or twisting your neck to the side can lead to surprising issues, like tight hamstrings or chronic back pain.

Almost everything starts at the spine. The strain caused by poor alignment builds over time, triggering discomfort and dysfunction throughout your body. Every chance to look up instead of down—or worse, down and to the side—helps realign your spine and protects against long-term damage.

These small, simple changes might feel inconvenient at first, but they're far less inconvenient than living with chronic pain.

A Story From the Clinic: The Power of a Gooseneck iPad Holder

While I was working in the clinic, I started asking all my neck pain clients about their daily habits because of the common trends I was noticing. One thing stood out: most of them used an iPad on their lap and on the couch. I recommended a gooseneck iPad holder to several clients, and the results were undeniable. The ones who were compliant and used it got significantly better quicker, and stayed better. This simple tool made such a profound difference that it sparked a realization: we need to go into people's homes and see what they're actually doing. If something as simple as a gooseneck holder could have such a big impact, what other small adjustments might be game changers?

The Fix is Simple. At the bare minimum RAISE YOUR DEVICE. Every degree higher matters. Your phone should be at eye level, no exceptions!

Tools like phone holders, gooseneck iPad stands, laptop stands, or adjustable monitor arms can make these adjustments effortless. Adding a phone holder to your desk or lifting papers to eye level to read can drastically reduce the time you spend looking down or twisting your neck. Every second counts, remember it all adds up over our lifetime! People often think I'm taking pictures when I hold my phone up in public. The truth? I'm saving my spine, ensuring that I can live pain-free for decades to come.

Beyond the Quick Fix

We've learned that treating neck pain isn't about finding a magical cure or the perfect posture. Instead, it's about:

- Understanding how daily habits impact your entire body
- Recognizing that movement, not stillness, is often the answer
- Making small, sustainable changes that add up to significant relief
- Viewing your body as an interconnected system rather than isolated parts

The Power of Awareness

Just as a blind person naturally expresses universal body language, your body carries innate wisdom about movement and posture. The key isn't forcing yourself into "perfect" positions, but rather:

- Creating a dynamic, varied approach to movement
- Listening to your body's signals
- Adapting your environment to support natural alignment
- Understanding that your next posture is your best posture

Your Path Forward

Remember that lasting relief doesn't come from temporary fixes or perfect postures. It comes from:

- Understanding the interconnected nature of your body
- Making mindful choices about how you move and position yourself
- Creating environments that support natural alignment
- Embracing movement as medicine

The solution to neck pain often lies not in what we add to our lives – more treatments, more medications, more procedures – but in what we modify in our daily habits. Your body has a remarkable capacity to heal when you give it the right conditions to do so. Every movement matters, every habit counts, and every small change brings you one step closer to lasting relief. Your pain-free future isn't about perfection – it's about progression, one mindful movement at a time.

Chapter 4
Wrist Whispers

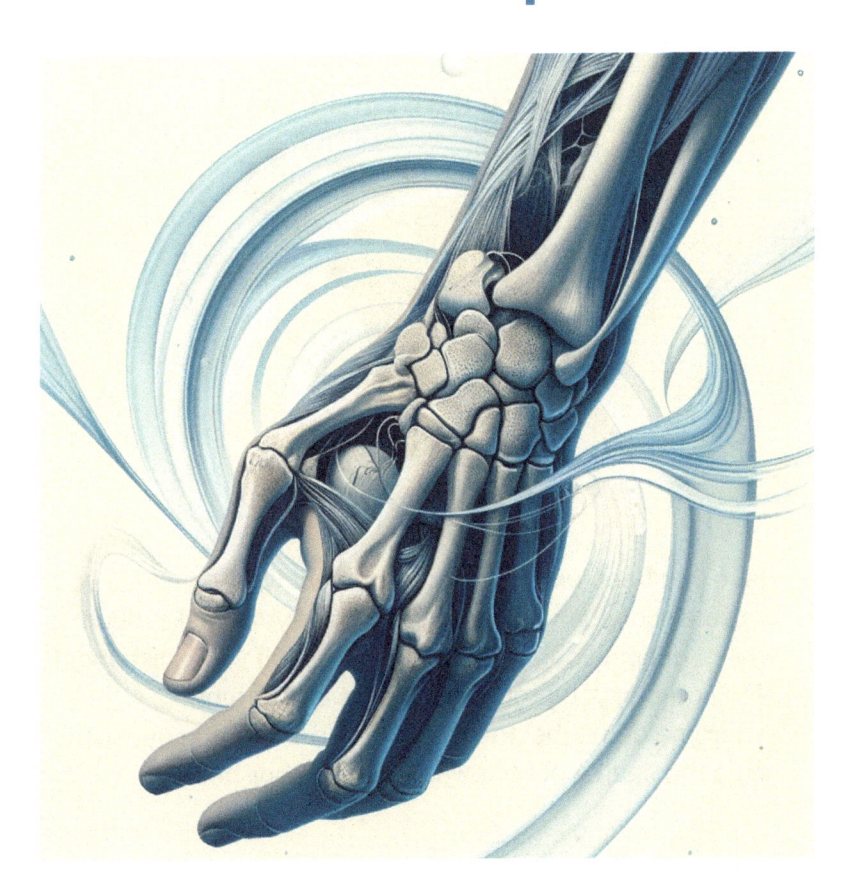

Wrist Whispers

Is Your Wrist Pain Really Just About Your Wrist?

Do You Have Wrist Pain?

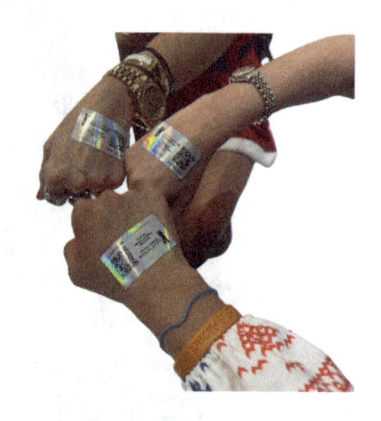

Have you been experiencing persistent wrist pain? Do you notice discomfort while performing everyday tasks, such as typing, gripping objects, or even at rest? If you're like most of my clients, you probably think it's carpal tunnel syndrome or maybe arthritis. Here's a surprising question: could the source of your wrist pain be your **neck**?

This may surprise you, many of our clients come to us thinking their wrist is the problem, only to discover that their cervical spine—the neck—is the source of their discomfort. Many people overlook the fact that nerve impingements or misalignments in the cervical spine can refer pain down the arm, manifesting in the wrist, hand, or even fingers.

This is called cervical radiculopathy, and it's more common than you might think. Many patients with wrist pain are misdiagnosed with carpal tunnel syndrome or arthritis when, in reality, the pain is referred from the neck. That's why the Slight Motion Method says: *Always rule out the spine first.*

According to a study in the Journal of Hand Surgery, a review of thousands of medically confirmed carpal tunnel syndrome cases showed that over 90% of patients examined also had a problem with the cervical nerves supplying the median nerve of the wrist.[3]

Often, wrist pain isn't just about repetitive hand movements—it's tied to poor posture and habits. Misalignment in the neck creates tension along the fascial lines that connect your neck, shoulders, and arms. If the nerves in your neck are irritated, they can send pain signals down the arm into the wrist and fingers, mimicking localized wrist issues.

Yes, your neck. Let me tell you about Sarah, an 83-year-old golfer who discovered this the hard way.

Sarah's Golf Story: When "Just Arthritis" Isn't the Answer

For many people, wrist pain is simply something to tolerate, especially as they age. Sarah, an avid golfer in her 80s, was told her wrist pain was due to "just arthritis." But Sarah's case had more to do with daily habits than with age or joint wear and tear. Her journey back to the golf course became one of the most valuable lessons I've learned about wrist pain.

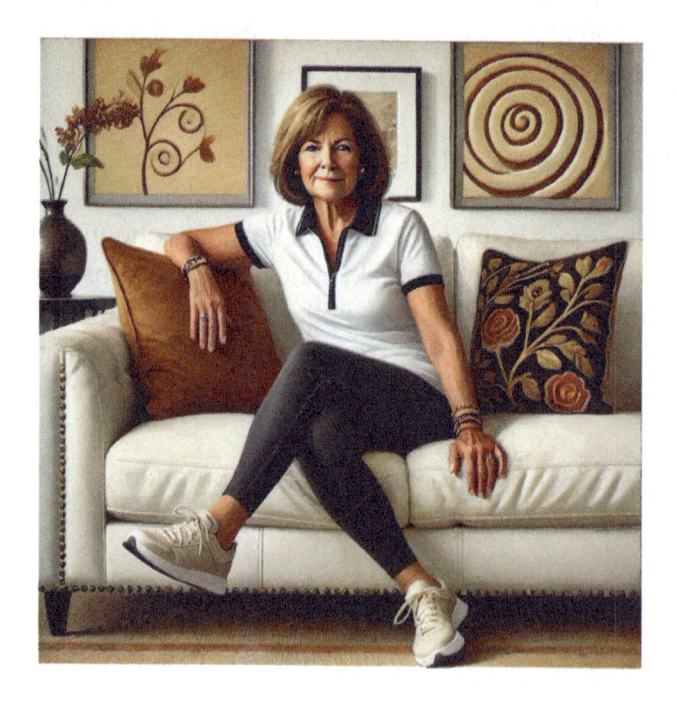

Sarah, an 83-year-old woman who came to me nearly in tears. She'd recently given up golf – her passion for over forty years – because she could no longer grip her club. Every doctor she'd seen had the same response: "It's arthritis. It's your age. There's nothing we can do."

But something didn't add up. When I visited her home, I noticed how she spent her downtime: perched on the side of her couch, right arm resting on the armrest, head tilted down and to the side as she scrolled through photos of her grandkids on her phone. "How long do you sit like this?" I asked. "Oh, just about 30 minutes a day," she replied, surprised by my interest in such a seemingly innocent habit.

Those 30 minutes were enough to throw off her entire body alignment. The way she rested her arm was causing her to lean and cause spine shifting. The head tilt was compressing nerves in her neck that affected her grip strength. It wasn't arthritis at all – it was her daily habits.

After adjusting her posture and making some simple changes to how she used her phone, Sarah's grip strength returned. A week later, she was back on the golf course. "My friends can't believe it," she told me. "They all thought I was done with golf forever."

The nerves that supply strength to your hand pass through the neck, and even small neck misalignments from head tilting can reduce their function. Consider your own posture when watching TV or using your phone.

Sarah's case is not unique. I often see patients who have been told their pain is simply 'arthritis' or 'age,' overlooking how posture habits play a central role.

Try this: Sit in a chair, tilt your head slightly to one side as if looking at your phone, and notice the subtle pull on your neck. Now, imagine holding this posture daily. It becomes clear how easily small habits can create big changes.

In fact, studies show that even a slight tilt of the head can add up to 10 pounds of pressure on the cervical spine, which over time affects the nerves controlling grip strength.[4]

Sarah's story demonstrates how common asymptomatic joint changes can be with age and why they don't always lead to pain. Studies estimate that as many as 50% or more of those with hand osteoarthritis show no symptoms.[5] This reinforces a key idea. While joint degeneration may be inevitable with age, focusing on daily habits—like posture, phone use, and seating positions—can often have a greater impact on managing and preventing symptoms than the joint changes themselves.

Sarah's story is a testament to how small changes, like adjusting posture for just a few minutes, can restore function—and remind us all to examine our daily habits a little closer.

While age-related changes in hand strength are real, research shows:

- Grip strength is a great indicator of overall health[6]
- Neural pathways remain adaptable throughout life
- Most age-related decline is actually related to lack of use

You're never too old to get better. If you have wrist pain, consider your neck as a potential source!

The Poker Player's Hidden Pattern: When Small Habits Create Big Problems

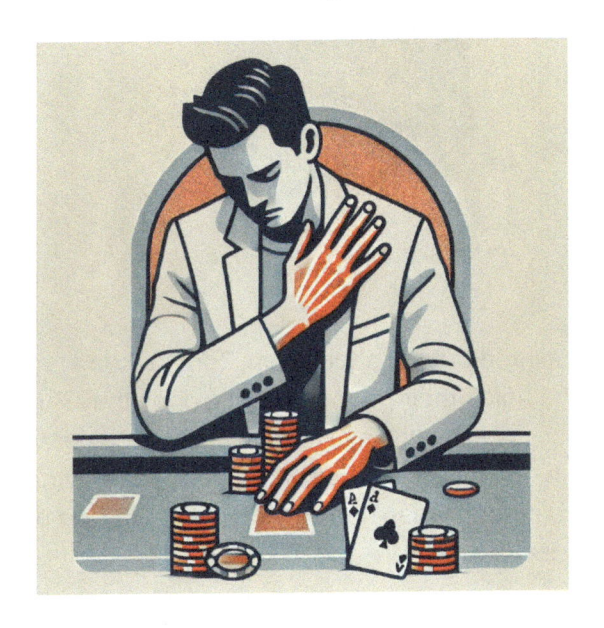

I'll never forget a poker game in San Francisco. I was sitting next to a guy who asked what I did for work. When he asked what made me different and how I fixed people so rapidly I explained it's all in the habits. He said can you give me an example? I looked over to a guy 2 seats over and said I'll bet ya one dollar he has hand pain. The guy said we should ask. So we did.

Tom responded yes how did you know? He reported he'd already had 2 cortisone injections and was considering a third, or possibly a surgery if it didn't improve. Multiple doctors had treated him, but the pain kept returning. Like many cases I see, everyone was focused on treating the symptom while missing the cause hiding in plain sight.

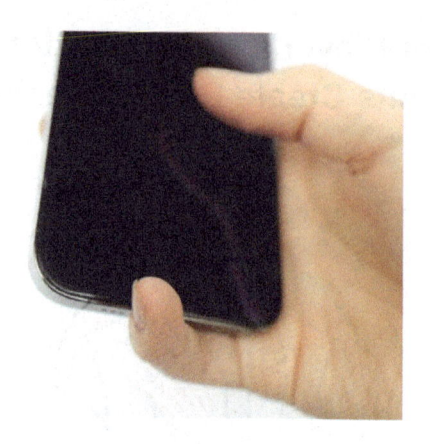

When I pointed out his phone grip, Tom looked startled. "Everyone holds their phone like this, don't they?" he asked. This is exactly why we're seeing an epidemic of hand pain – what seems normal isn't necessarily natural. The human hand wasn't designed for the way we use modern devices.

What made Tom's case particularly interesting was how this pattern repeated throughout his day. A week later he texted me he realized he was doing the same thing with his books – either propping them on his pinky or holding them from the side with his pointer finger. These seemingly innocent habits were creating a cumulative stress pattern.

"But it's just a few ounces," Tom protested when I explained the connection. What he didn't realize was that it's not just about weight – it's about duration and repetition. Studies show that sustained pressure on nerves, even if relatively mild, can cause more problems than brief periods of stronger pressure.

Try this:

Hold your phone normally for a moment. Now, notice your pinky position. If it's under the phone, you're asking that small finger to support about 200 grams of weight. Now multiply that by how many hours you spend on your phone each day. Starting to see the pattern?

After showing Tom how to modify his habits – *using a phone stand, alternating hands while reading, and being mindful of his grip patterns* – the change was remarkable. The persistent pain he'd been fighting for months began to subside.

"The strangest part," Tom told me later, "is that no one ever asked about how I held my phone or books. They just kept treating the pain." His experience reflects a broader pattern - treating symptoms without addressing habits rarely leads to lasting relief. A few weeks later, Tom was pain-free and had developed new awareness of his hand positions. His success wasn't unusual. We've seen it over and over again.

The pain we feel often has more to do with our daily habits than any underlying condition. For Tom, like many others, the solution wasn't in treating the symptom – it was in recognizing and adjusting the patterns that created it.

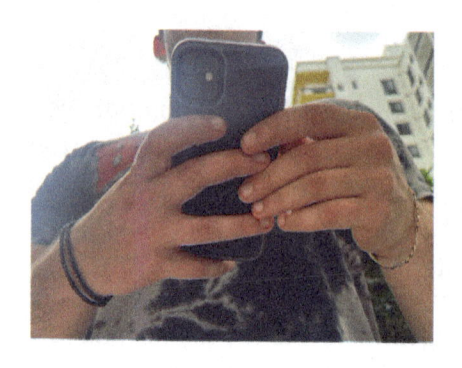

The telltale position I'd seen hundreds of times before: his pinky finger automatically sliding under the phone's base like a tiny kickstand. When we use our pinky as a phone support, we're asking the smallest, weakest finger to bear sustained weight in an unnatural position.

Research shows that this position can:

- Compress the ulnar nerve at Guyon's canal
- Create chronic strain in the hypothenar muscles
- Lead to altered hand biomechanics affecting overall grip strength
- Cause referral pain patterns throughout the hand and wrist

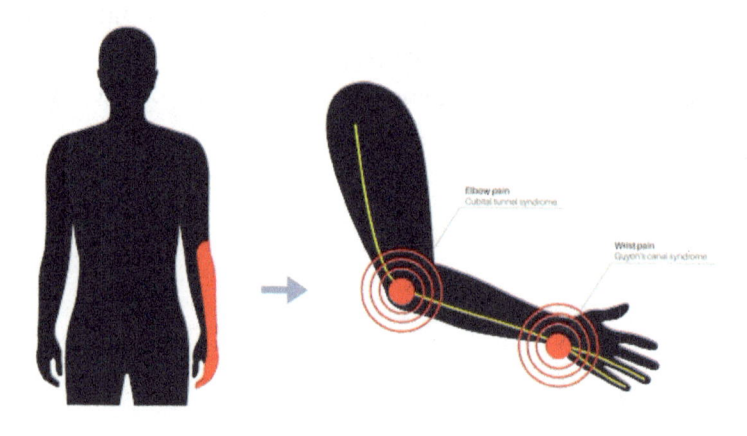

Tom's story reminds us that in our tech-focused world, we need to be more mindful of how we use our hands. The solution often isn't in treating the pain – it's in recognizing and adjusting the daily habits that created it in the first place. The most significant change wasn't just in Tom's hand health - it was in his understanding of how daily habits affect our bodies. "I used to think pain was something that just happened to you," he said. "Now I understand it's often something we accidentally do to ourselves through our habits."

How do you hold your phone? Do you put your pinky under it like a kickstand? Take a look at how you're holding your phone right now. How are you even holding this book? Even the way we hold our devices can cause numbness or tingling in hands/fingers.

Protect Your Pinkies! → **P.Y.P.**

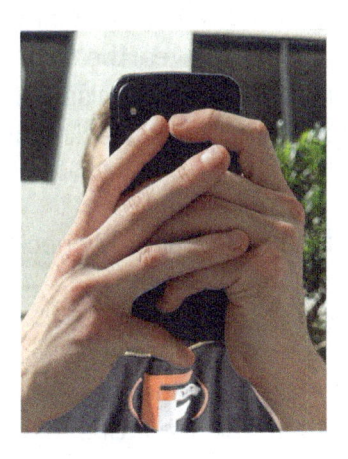

The Mysterious Middle Finger: A Back Pain Surprise

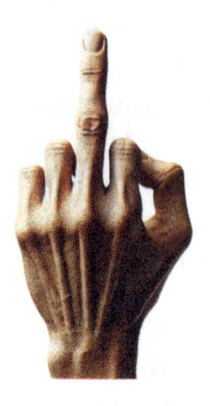

"My back hurts, but I guess I should mention something else..." Ashley said as our session was wrapping up. "My middle finger has been hurting for months. It's probably nothing related though, right?"

As a physical therapist, I've learned that these casual "by the way" comments often reveal the most important clues. Most practitioners might have dismissed this as a separate issue, but I had a hunch. "Let's check your neck," I suggested.

Ashley looked at me skeptically. "My neck? But the pain is in my finger."

What happened next left her speechless. After a quick screening of her neck, the finger pain that had bothered her for months simply vanished. She started calling me "the magician," but there was no magic involved – just an understanding of how our nervous system works.

The nerves that control sensation in your fingers run through your neck. When neck alignment is off, it can create pain that shows up far from the actual source.

I see this connection play out in different ways almost daily. Take Mark, a software developer who came to me with numbness in his thumb and index finger. He'd already bought an ergonomic keyboard and mouse, tried wrist braces, and even considered surgery. But when I watched him work, I noticed he constantly tucked his phone between his ear and shoulder while typing. This simple habit was compressing the nerves in his neck, causing his hand symptoms.

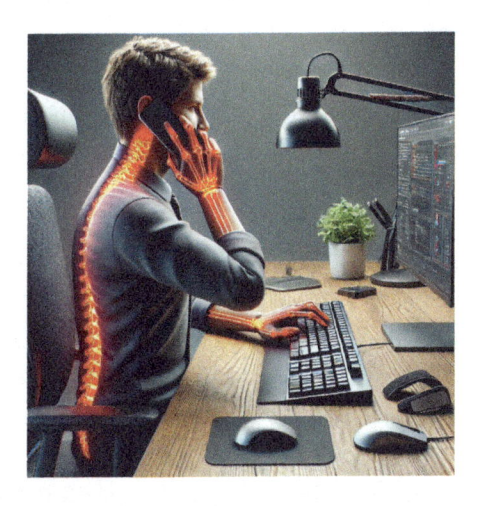

Or consider Janet, an artist who couldn't hold her paintbrush without pain. She'd been diagnosed with arthritis in her fingers, but during our session, I noticed she worked on her iPad for hours, holding it low in her lap and looking down. This position was straining her neck and affecting the nerve supply to her hands. Once we raised her iPad with a stand, her symptoms began to improve within days.

It's Not Always Where It Hurts: A Lesson From My Dad

The next story involves my own father after he fell off a ladder and broke his wrist, requiring surgery. The physical therapy he received focused solely on his wrist, which seemed logical at the time. However, he also had a few numb fingers, which his doctor assured him was "normal" due to the surgical procedure. But something wasn't adding up.

When I examined his arm, I touched his upper arm near the elbow, and he jumped. Pressing on specific spots near his elbow recreated the symptoms in his hand. The problem wasn't his wrist, it was the soft tissue near his elbow. After performing soft tissue mobilization to that area, he regained full feeling in his hand and fingers almost immediately.

This experience reinforced an important lesson. In a busy, high-paced clinical setting, it's easy to focus solely on the obvious injury while overlooking the rest of the patient. With limited time and many patients to see, the bigger picture can often get missed. However, true healing frequently lies beyond the apparent problem. By assessing the whole patient and their habits, rather than isolating treatment to one area, you can uncover the actual source of the issue and resolve it far more effectively. This holistic approach has become a cornerstone of my practice and the Slight Motion Method, ensuring that no underlying factors are ignored in the pursuit of lasting results.

The HF0 Experience: How Living and Learning Uncovered the Root of Pain

One of the most transformative periods in my career was at HF0, the world's most selective startup program. Over the past year, 27,000 teams began the application process, but only 10 are accepted into each batch. Those 10 teams move into a single house, where every aspect of their daily life is meticulously handled, leaving them free to focus entirely on their project.

That's where we come in. Our mission is to optimize their lives—right down to the smallest habit—so they can perform at their absolute best. HF0 believes the **Slight Motion Method** is essential to achieving that level of focus, efficiency, and success.

I spend several days every few months living and working closely with the founders. Immersing myself in their daily lives gave me a unique perspective on how our habits and environments create pain, and how to fix it efficiently. Observing their movements, work setups, and seemingly minor routines allowed me to connect the dots in ways traditional appointments often cannot. This experience was a cornerstone in shaping the principles behind this book.

One client I worked with there had been battling bilateral pinky numbness for over two years. He had consulted numerous experts and made countless adjustments to his workstation, swearing his setup was now perfect. Yet, the numbness persisted. After our first session, he reported feeling some improvement, his right pinky was better than his left, but both were still bothering him.

This detail piqued my curiosity: Why would one side improve faster than the other?

When I finally caught up with him the next day, I asked where he had been. He mentioned a long meeting in his room, which prompted me to take a closer look at his desk setup. At first glance, everything seemed fine. He had a wrist pad, a laptop stand, and what he believed to be an ergonomic setup. But as I watched him work, the root of the problem became clear.

The laptop stand wasn't high enough, and the keyboard and monitor were positioned too far away. This forced him to lean forward, placing constant pressure on the wrist pad and compressing the nerves in his wrists. His right side improved faster simply because it moved to operate the mouse, while his left remained static, bearing the brunt of the compression.

By making a few small adjustments like raising the laptop stand, bringing the keyboard closer, and encouraging him to be more mindful of his posture, his numbness began to resolve. Within days, he was symptom-free.

This case reinforced a critical insight that is the entire concept behind this book. We often unknowingly create our own pain through small, repeated actions in our daily routines. The solution isn't just about adding tools or treatments, it's about uncovering and eliminating these hidden stressors. My time at *HF0* taught me how to observe these patterns and identify the simplest, most effective fixes.

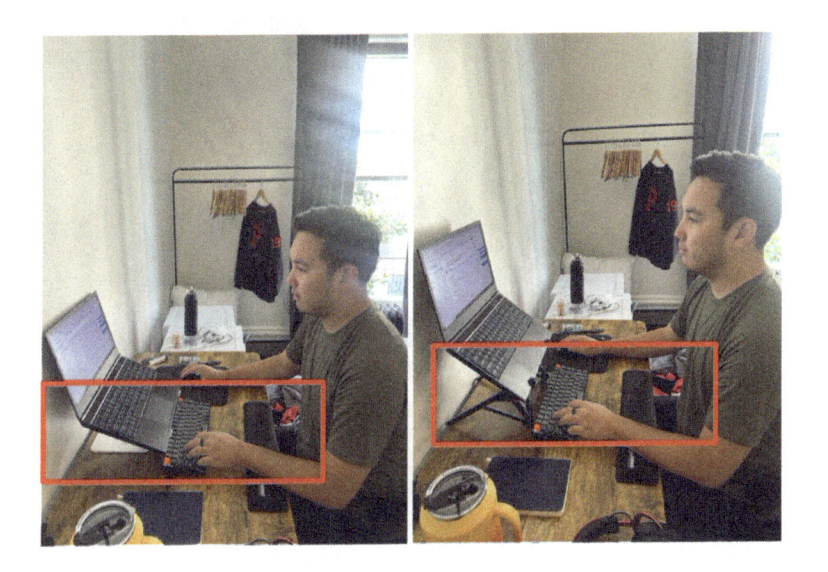

On the left image, the laptop is a little *too low* and his keyboard a *little too far away* for his long zoom meetings. This leads him to lean forward and compress the nerve that travels through the arm (ulnar nerve). The wrist pad made it easier to tolerate this position for longer periods. A slight adjustment to monitor height, bringing the keyboard closer, and awareness led to the bilateral pinky numbness mystery dissipating.

Think of your nerves like garden hoses running from your neck down your arms to your fingers. Just as a kinked hose reduces water flow, a compressed nerve from poor neck positioning can reduce proper signal transmission to your hands and fingers.

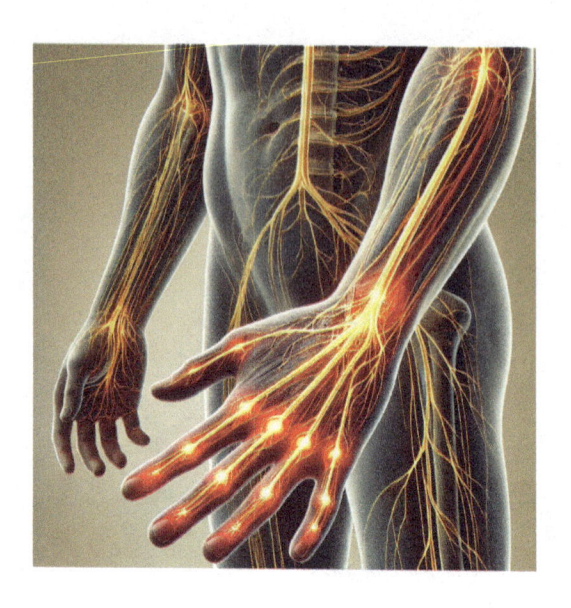

This can feel like:

- Unexplained pain in specific fingers
- Numbness or tingling in your hands
- Reduced grip strength
- Sharp or burning sensations
- Morning stiffness in your fingers

Try this simple test: Sit normally and notice if you have any hand or finger discomfort. Now, adjust your neck position by gently tucking your chin (think about making a slight double chin). Hold this for 30 seconds. Many people notice immediate changes in their hand symptoms.

"But it's just my finger hurting," you might say. Remember Ashley's story. Her middle finger pain wasn't a finger problem at all – it was her body's way of signaling that something needed attention higher up in the chain.

I've seen this pattern hundreds of times: A writer with wrist pain who worked with her laptop on the couch. A retiree with hand weakness who spent hours looking down at his crossword puzzles. A teenager with finger numbness who was constantly gaming on her phone. In each case, addressing their neck position made a dramatic difference in their hand symptoms.

The next time you experience hand or finger pain, don't immediately assume the problem is where you feel it. Take a moment to consider your daily habits. How do you hold your phone? Where do you position your tablet? How do you sit when working or relaxing? Sometimes the answer lies in the most unexpected places – like a magic trick that isn't really magic at all.

Set a reminder on your phone to check your neck position every hour. Are you looking down at a device? Is your head tilted to one side? Small adjustments in neck position throughout the day can make a big difference in hand and finger symptoms. This is a perfect example of how crucial it is to address the neck whenever there's wrist, hand, or finger pain. Often, the nerve pathways that run through the neck are the real culprits, causing symptoms to show up in other areas of the body.

Emma's Story: The iPad, The Bed, and The Mysterious Hand Swelling

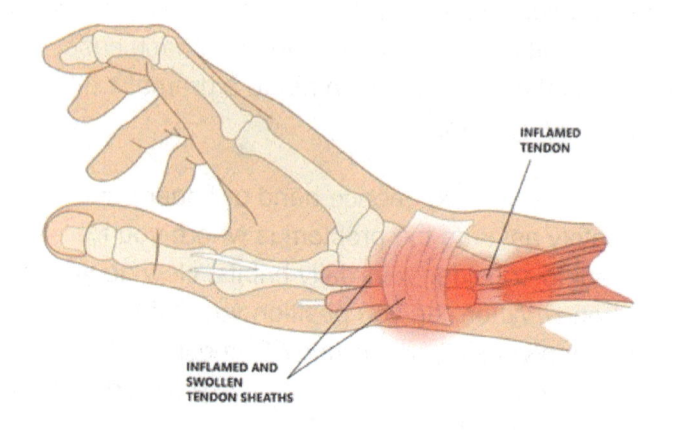

Emma loved nothing more than getting lost in a good book. An avid reader who came to me with severe wrist pain and swelling that her doctor had diagnosed as *De Quervain's tenosynovitis*. This is a condition where the tendons on the thumb side of your wrist become inflamed, causing pain and swelling. This often happens with repetitive movements like texting, scrolling, or typing. She'd already tried anti-inflammatory medications and was considering surgery. "I don't understand," she said. "I've always been a reader. Why is this happening now all of a sudden?"

The clue came when I visited her at home. Emma had recently switched from physical books to an iPad, which she used while propped up in her adjustable bed. For hours each day, she'd lie there holding the device, her wrists bent at awkward angles to keep the screen stable. "But I'm so comfortable," she protested when I pointed this out. "And I love that I can read in the dark!"

That "comfortable" position, combined with the iPad's weight, was straining the tendons in her thumb and wrist. The propped-up position in bed was doubly problematic – it was affecting both her neck alignment and her wrist position.

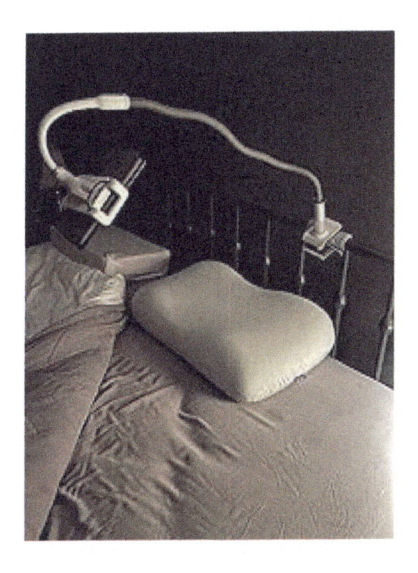

We made two simple changes: first, we got her a gooseneck tablet holder that could attach to her bedside table. Second, we adjusted her reading position to support better spine alignment. Within two weeks, her swelling decreased significantly. A month later, she called to cancel her surgical consultation.

Sometimes our favorite "comfortable" positions are the very ones causing our pain. Modern conveniences like tablets can create new stresses on our bodies that traditional books didn't. What feels comfortable in the moment can mask slowly developing problems. Modern conveniences often require modern solutions to protect our bodies.

That comfort was deceptive. The iPad's weight, though minimal, required her thumbs and wrists to maintain constant tension. Combined with her propped-up position, it was creating a perfect storm of strain on her tendons.

Emma's story teaches us that even the most relaxing activities, when done in an unnatural position, can strain our bodies. Small changes, like using a tablet holder or changing posture every so often, allowed her to read comfortably again. Sometimes comfort is about finding sustainable positions that work with our bodies. With these small adjustments to her setup, Emma was able to continue her favorite hobby pain-free. This story shows how simple changes in how we hold and position devices can prevent strain, proving that these "comfortable" positions may not be as ergonomic as we think.

Triggered By A Laptop on the Lap

Maria, a remote worker, developed trigger finger and received a cortisone shot. The pain improved temporarily but returned months later. When she called for another injection, the scheduler wasn't surprised – they'd already penciled her in for regular shots every few months saying "Wow yours lasted longer than others."

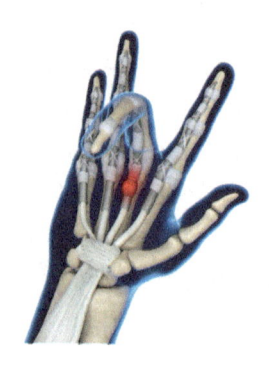

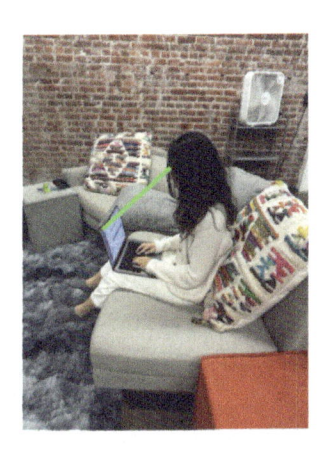

But before she got that second shot, we looked at her work setup. She was spending hours on her laptop while lounging on her couch. No wonder the cortisone wore off – she was recreating the problem daily. After setting up a proper workstation with a laptop stand and no couch work, her pain disappeared completely. She canceled that second shot and hasn't needed one since.

Is Your Office Setup to Blame for Your Wrist Pain?

When an ergonomic upgrade backfired

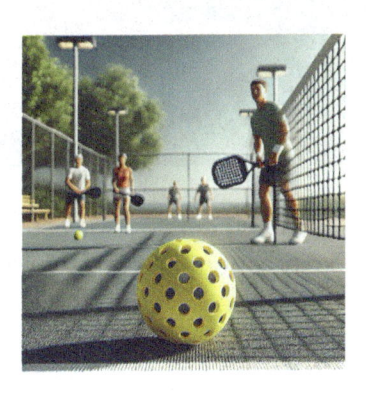

Jake consulted me because his wrist was bothering him during pickleball. "I've been playing pickleball for years without any issues," he said, demonstrating how his backhand was now causing pain.

"But lately, I can barely get through a game."

As we went through his daily habits, nothing unusual stood out. He hadn't changed his racket or technique. Then he casually mentioned his company's recent ergonomic upgrade program.

"Wait," I said, "when did you get the new mouse?"

Jake pulled up his email to check the date. His face suddenly lit up with realization – the wrist pain had started just days after switching to his new "ergonomic" mouse. The pain wasn't just affecting his computer work; it was carrying over into his pickleball game. Such a simple change at work was affecting his life outside the office.

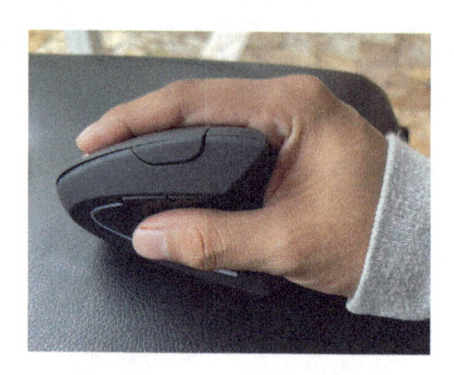

We immediately switched him to a vertical mouse, which positions the hand in a more functional and "handshake" position. Within a few weeks, not only could he work comfortably, but his pickleball game was back to normal.

This case taught me something important about mouse use. Variety can be more beneficial than finding the "perfect" mouse. Now I often recommend using two different ones throughout the day – one mouse before lunch, a different mouse after lunch. Think of it like a workout for your wrist rather than a repetitive stress injury. Instead of doing the same movement hundreds of times a day, you're training different muscle groups and movement patterns.

Small changes in our tools can have big effects on our bodies, even affecting the activities we love outside of work. Sometimes the best solution isn't finding one perfect setup, but creating healthy variety in our movements. Could you use your other hand at times?

The Tale of Two Heights: A Workspace Mystery

How Is Your Keyboard and Mouse Positioned? Take a look at your desk setup. Is your keyboard at one height and your mouse at another?

Andres consulted me after two cortisone shots in his wrist. His pain was so severe he was considering surgery. When I visited his office, I noticed something peculiar – his keyboard was tucked away in a cubby under his desk, while his mouse sat on top of the desk. Every time he needed to use the mouse, he had to pull his arm back then reach over and up, creating an awkward angle in his wrist.

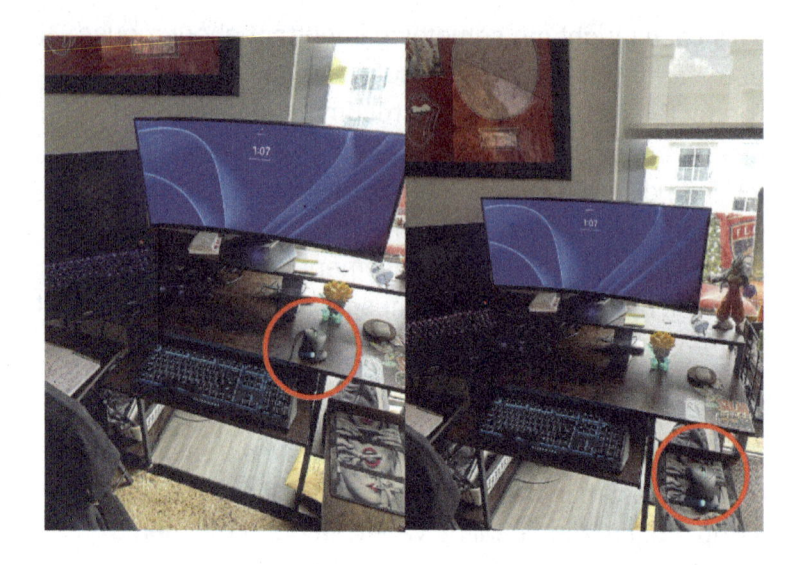

Andres wanted to understand why his wrist pain had become so persistent. After discussing his routine, we realized he plays a lot of pickleball and likely sustained a slight strain or overuse injury there. This minor issue was being continuously aggravated and prolonged by the misaligned setup at his desk, turning a small problem into a chronic one.

Following the Slight Motion Method and simply aligning his keyboard and mouse at the same height resolved his pain within weeks. Misalignments that seem minor often create a ripple effect of strain, especially when combined with other stressors like sports or repetitive tasks.

Keyboards

When it comes to typing, avoid using your laptop's built-in keyboard. This setup can create constant internal shoulder rotation, increasing the risk of impingement, especially in the arm that frequently uses the trackpad.

Additionally, your laptop should ideally be on a stand to bring the screen to eye level. Pair it with an external mouse and keyboard to maintain proper posture and minimize strain on your shoulders and wrists.

Have You Tried a Split Keyboard?

A split keyboard can reduce wrist strain by allowing your hands to rest in a more natural position. If you haven't tried one yet, it might be a simple solution to your wrist pain.

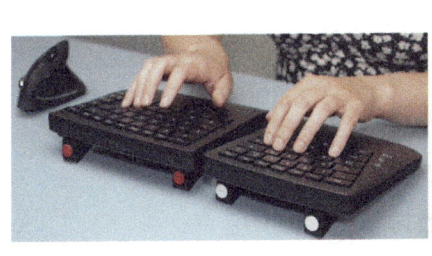

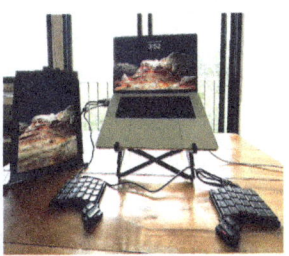

Questions to Ask Yourself:

- Have you recently changed any part of your work setup?
- Are you using the same mouse position all day?
- Is pain from work affecting your hobbies or activities?
- Could you introduce more variety in your movements?

Practical Solutions

Every inch you raise your phone exponentially reduces the strain on your spine.

Try these:

- **The Eye-Level Rule:** Hold your phone at eye level for essential tasks
- **The Elbow Support:** Rest your elbows on a table or armrest to help hold your phone higher
- **The 20-20-20 Rule:** Every 20 minutes, look at something 20 feet away for 20 seconds
- **Voice Commands:** Use voice-to-text for longer messages
- **Phone Stand:** Invest in a stand for your desk or table

Solving the Real Problem

Pain isn't always what it seems. Whether it's wrist pain, numb fingers, or unexplained discomfort, the true cause often lies far from where the symptoms appear. From desk setups and posture habits to overlooked injuries and repetitive strain, small hidden patterns in our daily lives can lead to big problems.

The good news? Small, intentional changes can also provide big relief. By stepping back, assessing the whole body, and looking beyond the obvious, we can uncover the root causes of pain and address them efficiently. The Slight Motion Method isn't about quick fixes. It's about understanding how our habits, environments, and movements shape our bodies and making adjustments that truly last. So the next time you feel pain, ask yourself: is this really where the problem is coming from?

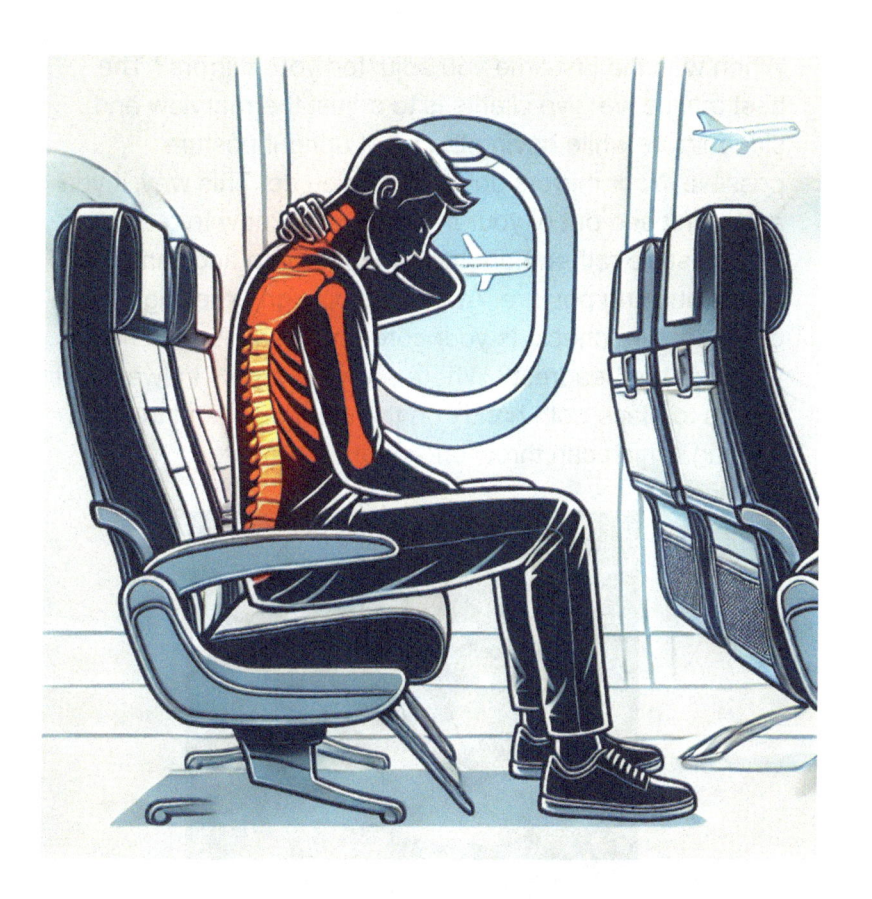

Chapter 5
Transportation Troubles

Transportation Troubles

Do Your Transportation Habits Affect Your Neck?

How Do You Sit While Driving?

When was the last time you adjusted your mirrors? The best advice we give clients is to adjust the rearview and side mirrors while having the most upright posture possible. Your mirrors don't move, you do. This way, if you ever can't see out of your mirrors, you'll know to readjust your posture rather than move the mirror to accommodate your slouching posture. At every stop sign or red light, do a quick posture check: Is your core engaged? Is your head touching the headrest? Where are your arms? I always tell clients to place both hands on the steering wheel to avoid leaning, which can throw off spinal alignment.

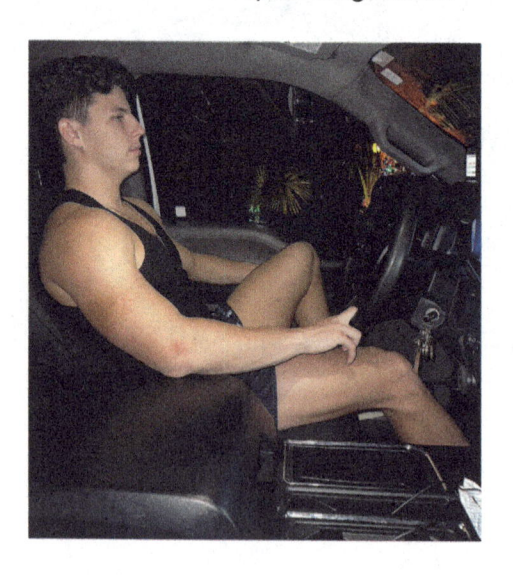

Are you sitting on your tailbone or your butt cheeks while driving? Many of us unknowingly slouch onto our tailbones, which can lead to lower back pain. Sit up tall and tighten your core—it will slightly rotate your pelvis forward, positioning you on your butt cheeks and aligning your spine. This small adjustment can make a big difference in reducing strain during long drives.

When's the last time you adjusted your car seat? Most people say never. Ideally, you should move it every 20 minutes. At red lights, adjust it up, down, forward, or backward. Everything in life that moves needs to move. These subtle shifts help keep your body from stiffening up and encourage improved blood flow.

The Leaning Society – Is It Hurting Your Spine?

In today's world, we've become a society of leaners. How often do you see someone lying on their side while watching TV, propping themselves up with one arm? Or placing a pillow under their side while lying down? Why do we lean so much? Probably because of underlying weaknesses and our bodies crave external support. These positions are tough on the spine and are one of the reasons scoliosis is so common. We tend to mimic the postures we see in our families growing up, and poor habits can be passed down without us even realizing it.

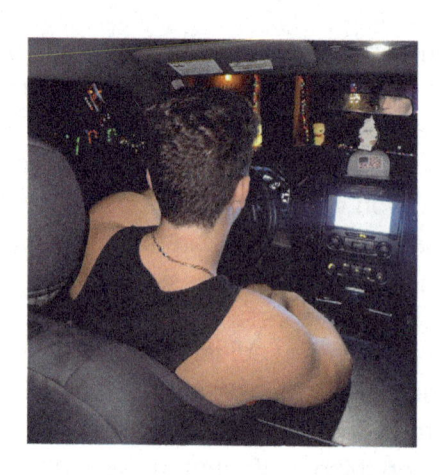

Do you put one hand or two hands on the steering wheel? Have you ever caught yourself leaning to one side when you drive, resting an arm on the console or window? This subtle shift can misalign your spine and pelvis.

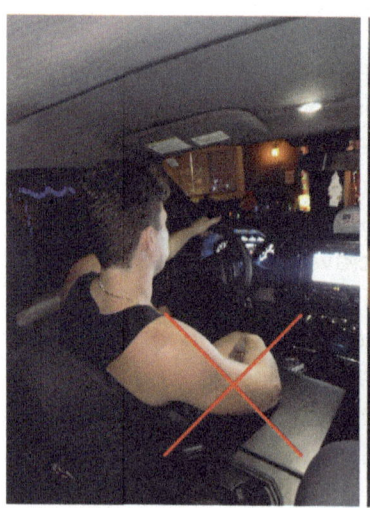

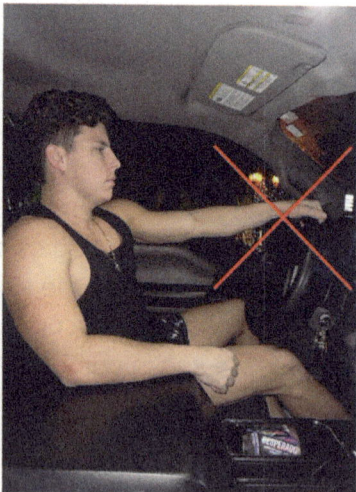

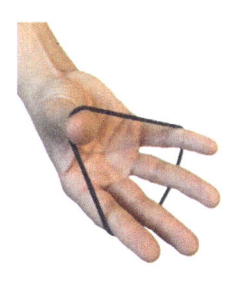

A quick trick I suggest is keeping a hair tie on your wrist to play with as a replacement for leaning. Choose anything to fidget with to help avoid leaning.

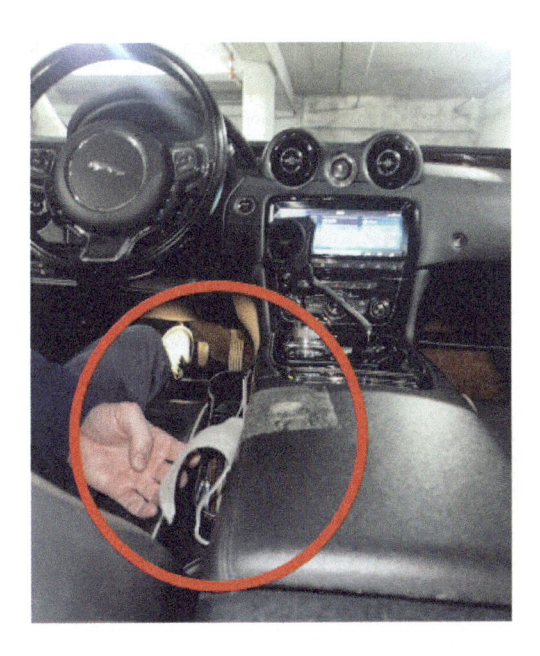

Take a look around your car. Are there signs of wear and tear from your habits? Is your center console scuffed or worn down in certain spots from constant leaning? These visible clues can reveal how ingrained certain postures have become in your daily life. Noticing these patterns is the first step to correcting them.

The Tesla Troubles: A Case of Misplaced Blame

Elon was ready to give up. "I can't drive this car anymore," he said as we stood in his driveway. "I've tried everything—seat cushions, backrests, even looked into replacing the seat entirely. Nothing helps. Every time I drive, my back kills me."

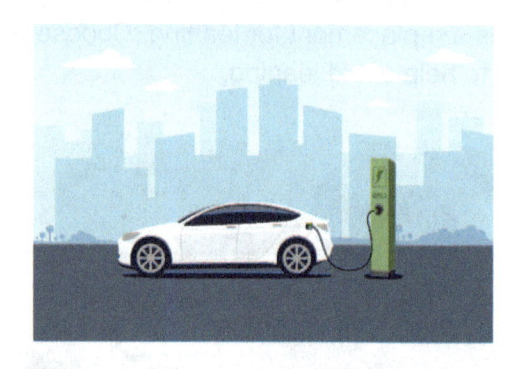

Elon had always been a fan of cutting-edge technology, and his new Tesla was no exception. But just a few months into ownership, he was ready to sell it, convinced the car itself was the problem.

"It has to be the seat design," he insisted.

Instead of offering a quick fix, I wanted to address the issue at its root. "Show me how you sit when you're driving," I said.

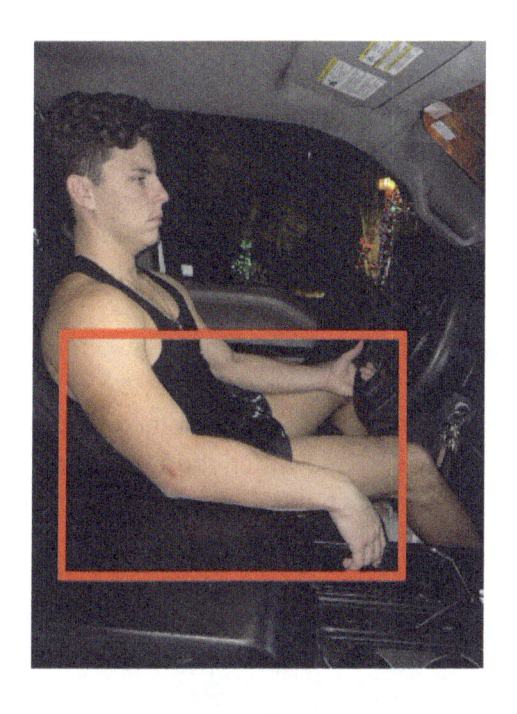

Elon got into the driver's seat, and it all became clear. He rested one elbow on his lap and the other on the center console, causing his spine to twist subtly, but significantly. This asymmetry was putting uneven pressure on his back, leading to his persistent pain.

"It's not the car," I explained. "It's how you're sitting in it."

Skeptical but willing to try, Elon followed my advice. Together, we adjusted his mirrors to encourage an upright posture, placed both hands on the wheel to eliminate leaning, and built in posture checks at every stoplight.

A week later, Elon called me, his tone completely different. "You're not going to believe this," he said. "I've been driving pain-free all week. I can't believe I was ready to sell my Tesla over something as simple as how I was sitting." By addressing the root cause, his driving posture, Elon not only kept his dream car but also eliminated the back and neck pain that had plagued him for months.

The Valet Driver's Syndrome

It's a familiar scene: I pull up to a hotel or restaurant, hand my keys to the valet, and watch them zip away with my car. But what's become just as familiar are the conversations that follow when I return.

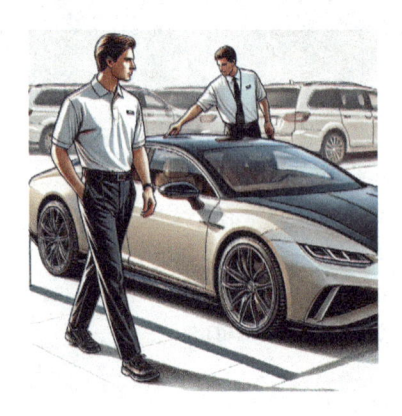

"Hey, doc," one valet said as he handed me back my keys, "Can I ask you something? My shoulder's been killing me lately."

It wasn't the first time. Over the years, countless valet drivers have stopped to ask me about shoulder pain. Whether it's at luxury hotels, downtown restaurants, or event venues, they all experience some type of pain.

"I'm not sure what I'm doing wrong," they'd say, wincing as they gestured to their shoulder. "I feel it every time I park cars. It's getting worse."

So, I started asking questions. "How do you typically hold the steering wheel? Are you using one hand or both? Do you notice if it's worse after making sharp turns?"

It didn't take long to identify the culprit: **The Valet Driver's Syndrome.**

Many valet drivers spend hours gripping the steering wheel with one hand, usually their dominant arm, while making repeated tight turns into parking spaces. The constant motion of cranking the wheel, often at awkward angles, puts immense strain on their shoulders.

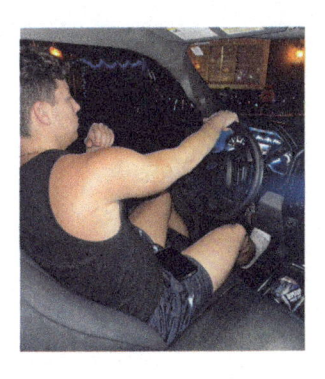

One valet driver demonstrated how he handled turns, his right hand firmly on the wheel as he swung into a tight left-hand turn. "See this?" I pointed out. "You're impinging your shoulder every time you do that. Since it's already irritated, you're making it worse with every repetition."

The solution wasn't to stop being a valet—it was to adjust their steering wheel grip and hand position.

Driving Ergonomics

- Lack of movement and asymmetrical postures (like one-arm propping) while driving can exacerbate back pain
- Adjusting your seat and mirror positions before you drive can help you notice and correct slouching
- A client eliminated pain by changing how he sat in his car, preventing uneven pressure

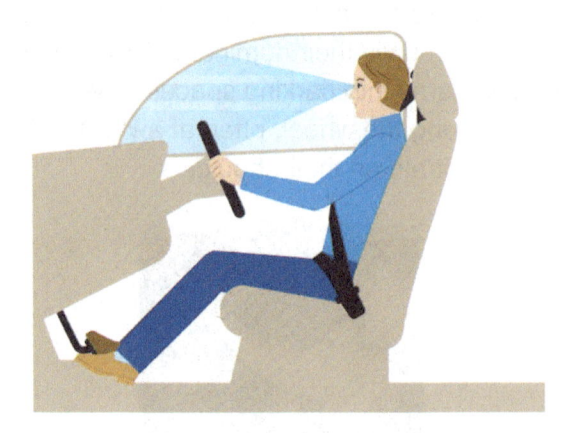

Do You Use Your Phone While You Drive?

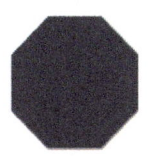

PSA
Stop Using Your Phone While You Drive!

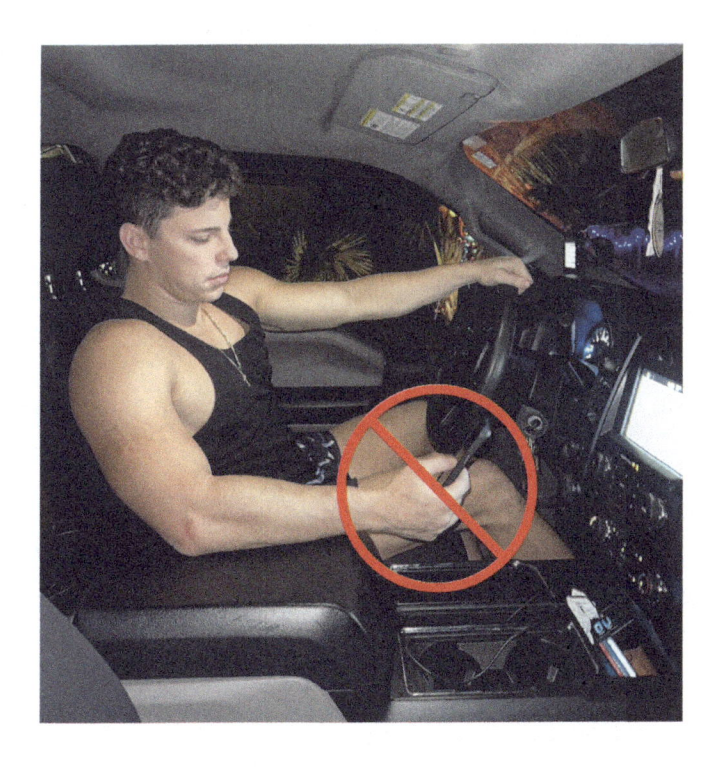

"The only thing worse than looking down, is looking DOWN & TO THE SIDE"

The Rainy Day That Revealed Everything

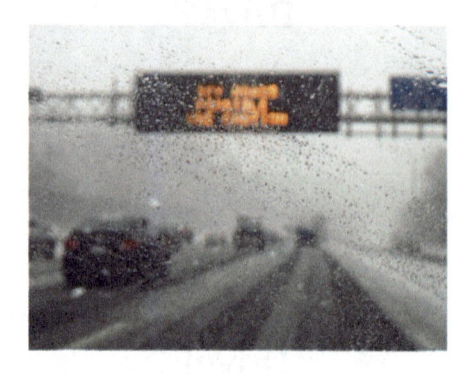

"I don't understand," Mark said, flexing his numb thumb. "I've had every test imaginable - carpal tunnel, nerve conduction, MRIs. Everything's normal, but this numbness won't go away." As a sales representative spending hours on the road, this mysterious symptom was affecting both his work and his peace of mind.

The breakthrough came unexpectedly during a torrential rainstorm that left him stuck in traffic for 45 minutes. The next day, his symptoms were dramatically worse. That's when I asked him to show me exactly how he sits in his car.

"Just normal driving," he demonstrated, immediately resting his left elbow on the door, his right hand loosely gripping the wheel at 4 o'clock. His spine subtly curved to the left to compensate.

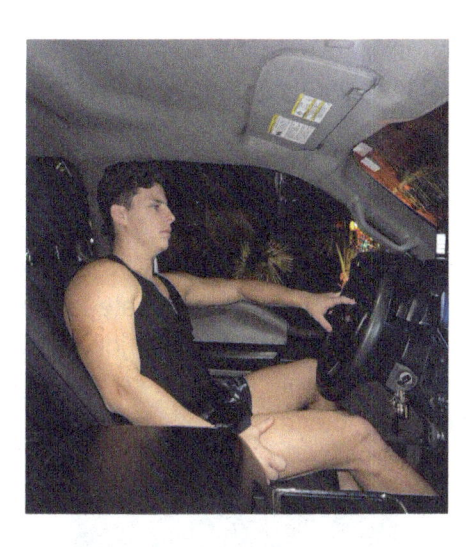

Think about Mark's typical position:

- Left elbow propped on window
- Single-handed steering
- Spine curved laterally
- Hours maintained in this position
- Neck compensating for asymmetry

"But it's comfortable," he protested when I explained how his casual driving position of resting his arm was affecting his nerve pathways.

We established a new driving protocol:

- Mirror positioned for optimal posture
- Both hands on wheel (except for necessary movements)
- Posture check at every red light
- Head in contact with the head rest
- Regular shoulder blade squeezes
- Core engagement reminders

Two weeks later, Mark's thumb sensation was improving. "I never realized how my casual driving position was affecting my whole body," he said.

"That rainstorm was actually a blessing in disguise."

Three months later, Mark had not only resolved his thumb numbness but had become an advocate for proper driving posture among his sales team. "They joke that I've become the posture police," he told me, "but several of them have noticed their own aches and pains improving."

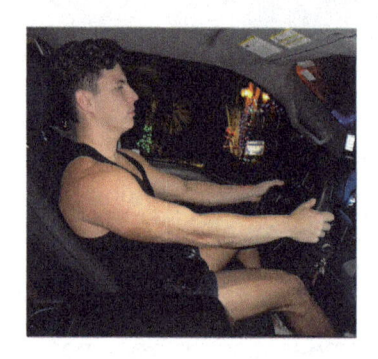

Take a "driving audit":

- Where do your elbows rest?
- How many hands on the wheel?
- Is your mirror set for better posture?
- What happens at stop lights?

Your driving position affects:

- Nerve pathways through neck and shoulders
- Spinal alignment
- Muscle tension
- Blood flow to upper extremities

Every minute in a better position is an investment in your body's well-being. As Mark learned, sometimes the route to healing starts with how we hold the steering wheel. Holding a static driving posture, such as leaning to one side with one arm on the window, causes uneven strain on the body. In Mark's case, this slight twist in his spine and shoulders was affecting his nerves and creating tension in his neck and shoulder, which manifested as numbness in his thumb. By aligning his body with both hands on the wheel and his head against the headrest, we ensured an even distribution of forces on both sides of his body. This balance helps reduce nerve compression and muscular tension, which directly alleviated his symptoms.

Steering Your Body: The Impact of How You Hold the Wheel

The way you hold the steering wheel can have a surprising impact on your body, especially during long drives. Gripping too tightly or positioning your arms too high can lead to tension in your shoulders, neck, and upper back, while slouching forward can exacerbate strain on the thoracic spine. Additionally, uneven hand placement can create imbalances, forcing one side of your body to compensate for the other.

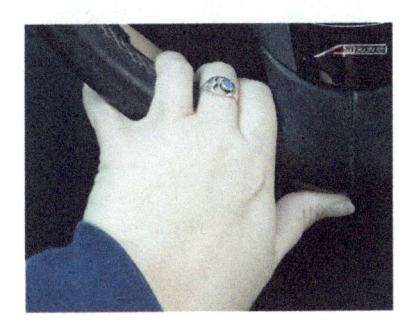

Over time, these habits can contribute to stiffness, discomfort, and even chronic pain. Adjusting your posture, relaxing your grip, and positioning your hands symmetrically on the wheel can help reduce these stresses and promote better alignment, making driving a more comfortable experience.

For optimal ergonomics, aim to position your hands at "9 and 3" or slightly lower, allowing your arms to rest comfortably with a slight bend at the elbows. Pair this with an upright seat position and ensure your shoulders are relaxed and not hunched. Small adjustments like these can prevent discomfort and help you stay more comfortable on long drives.

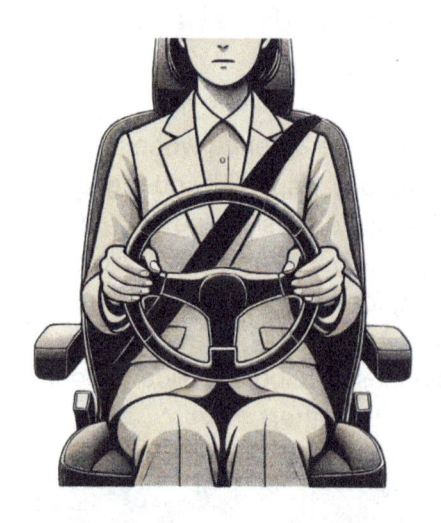

A Grandmother's Car Entry: The Simple Shift for Pain-Free Rides

Margaret was 72 years old when she came to see me, frustrated by hip pain that seemed worse after every car ride. "It's not even the driving that bothers me," she explained. "It's just getting in and out that's become a nightmare." An active grandmother who prided herself on her independence, she wasn't ready to give up her daily drives to see her grandchildren.

During our next session, I met her in her driveway. "Show me how you normally get into your car," I requested.

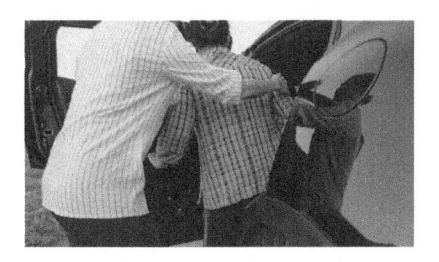

What I saw was a familiar pattern - one I see with many clients. Margaret approached her sedan from the side, lifted her right leg into the car while balancing on her left, then twisted and swung herself into the seat. Each entry was like a mini gymnastics routine, putting significant strain on her hip.

"I've always done it this way," she said, noticing my concerned expression. "Doesn't everyone?"

"Let me show you something I learned during my time in inpatient rehab facilities," I offered. "Actually, there's a gentler way," showing her a simple method I call the "sit-then-turn" technique, often taught in physical therapy.

- Back up to the seat until you feel it against your legs
- Slowly sit down while still facing out
- Then turn your body into the car, bringing your legs in last

Margaret looked skeptical. "That seems so... formal. Like something you'd do in physical therapy."

"Just try it once," I encouraged.

Her eyes widened as she completed the movement. "That felt... easier. Much easier actually."

"But I can't do this every time," Margaret protested. "Sometimes I'm in a hurry, or in a tight parking spot."

"What if you just tried this at home?" I suggested. "In your garage or driveway, where you have space and aren't rushed? With a little bit of practice, you'll build muscle memory, and soon it will feel natural to get in and out of the car without having to think about it."

Three weeks later, Margaret's hip pain had noticeably improved. "I thought you were being overly cautious," she admitted. "But just changing how I get in and out of the car at home has made such a difference. Sometimes I even find myself doing it in parking lots without thinking!"

The traditional way of entering a car forces:

- **Balancing on one leg,** adding stress to our joints, especially for those with hip or knee sensitivity.
- **Twisting while supporting body weight that can** strain hip and core muscles.
- **Lifting and swinging the legs simultaneously**, increasing pressure on the hip joint.

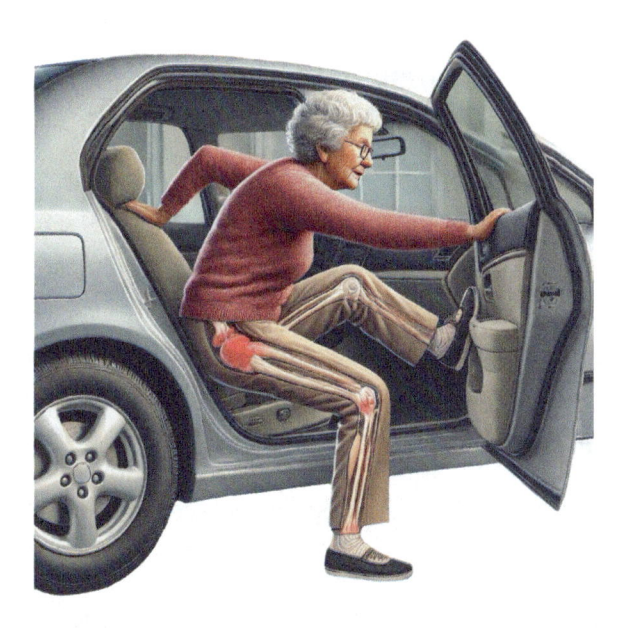

Do You Sit On Your Wallet?

If you sit on your wallet—or even a handkerchief—you're creating a problem that I can't fix and neither can a surgeon. Take a look around at people limping noticeably. Odds are, many of them have something in their back pocket they didn't bother removing before sitting down. It's not their fault; most people just don't know any better. But let me be clear: this is a *non-negotiable*.

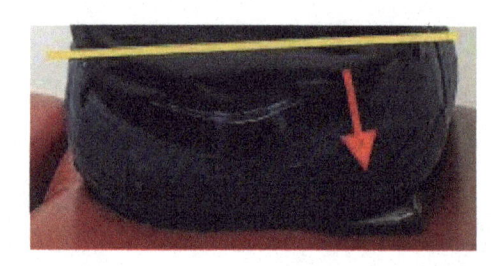

I'm so passionate about this issue that I've even brought it up at bars. If I see someone with a wallet in their back pocket, I'll strike up a conversation. The response? Almost everyone listens, and 99% of them admit they've dealt with chronic back pain, a hip or knee replacement, or other related issues.

When I was in San Francisco, I often used Uber to travel to clients with my table, and the drivers would inevitably ask me questions about their back or hip pain. Time and again, their stories were the same: they sat on their wallets, leaned to one side while driving, and slept without a pillow between their knees. Many had even undergone spine surgery without knowing their habits were a root cause of their issues.

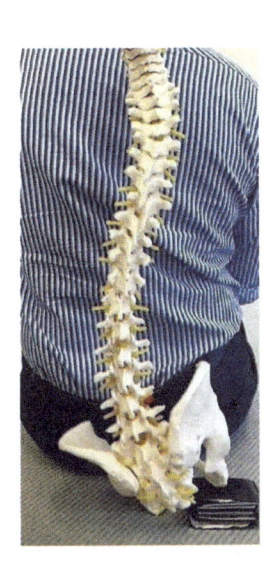

Here's the problem: sitting on your wallet causes a slight but constant shift in your spine. Think of it this way—if you put a credit card or small rock under your foot and walked around all day, you'd definitely notice it but you have all these muscles between your foot and spine that can shorten or lengthen. Now imagine that small, uneven pressure placed directly under your spine, without the cushion of muscles to absorb it. Over time, this subtle shift adds up, leading to chronic pain or even structural issues.

A wallet under your foot might be annoying, but your body can adapt to some extent. Put that same pressure near your spine, and there's no room for adaptation—just strain and misalignment. The result? A spine that shifts and strains with every movement offsetting all the jenga blocks.

If this sounds familiar, now is the time to change. Take the simple step of removing your wallet before you sit down. Your body will thank you, and you'll avoid joining the growing number of people suffering from preventable pain.

Do You Sleep on Planes, Trains or Buses?

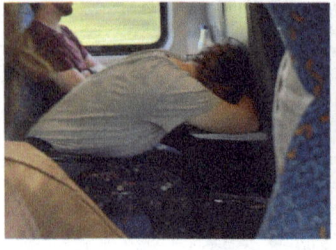

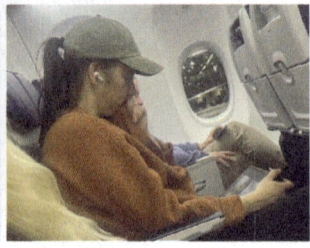

Do you fly or take long train rides more than once a month? How do you sleep during those trips? One of my clients flies twice a month for work, and she spends much of that time reading, scrolling on her phone, or trying to nap. If you're sleeping on a plane without proper neck support, like a neck pillow, you could be setting yourself up for major cervical pain. I've even given up sleeping in cars for the same reason—it's just not worth the pain that follows.

If you think about it even if you're only traveling twice a month this can be a major source of pain. You travel one day, the pain doesn't set in for 2-3 days and lasts about a week and then you're already traveling again!

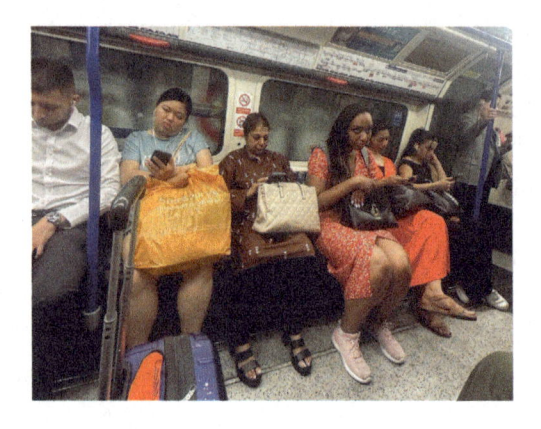

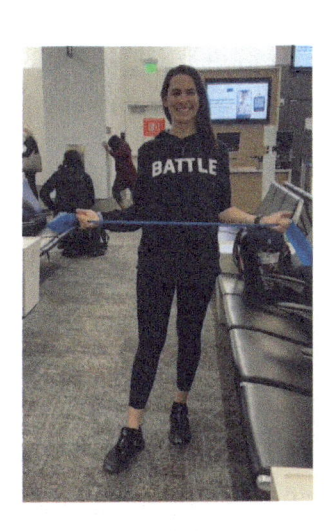

When I travel I always bring a resistance band and do some exercises while waiting to board. You have to be at the airport over an hour early, so you might as well get a workout in. Look around next time you're in the airport at how many people are spending more than 10 minutes looking straight down at their phones, or leaning on things, or using a laptop without a laptop stand.

Think about it—if you're a passenger, something as simple as using a neck pillow correctly or adjusting your posture can make a huge difference. Most people on a plane wear their neck pillow with the gap in front, but flipping it around works far better. Worn backwards, it functions more like a neck brace, providing proper support and preventing strain.

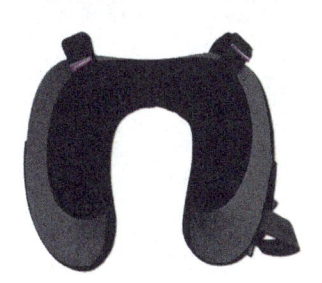

When we nap in cramped seats without neck support, the weight of our head, often tilted forward or to the side, strains the cervical spine. Even 10 minutes of leaning forward to check your phone can start to build up pressure in your neck. Over time, these habits cause what we think of as "mystery pain" that lingers long after the trip.

Small Changes, Big Impact

Take a moment to observe people next time you're in transit—many are hunched over their phones, leaning heavily on armrests, or working on laptops without any ergonomic support. All of these habits add up, especially if you're traveling regularly.

Try this next time you travel:

- Use a neck pillow!
    - Try turning the pillow around so the opening is in the back

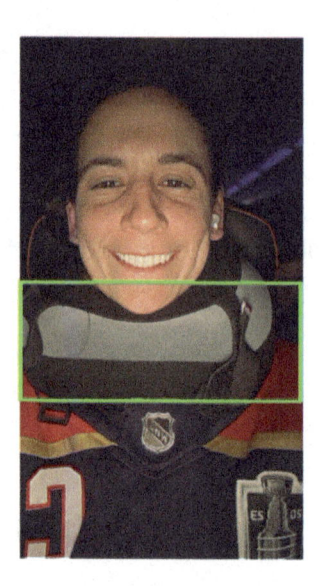

- Avoid leaning forward for extended periods to look at screens.
- Activate your muscles with a resistance band before boarding

Breaking the travel pain cycle often requires simple, proactive steps. Consider small posture adjustments and travel-friendly exercises to keep your neck and shoulders pain-free, no matter how often you're on the go.

Mindful Device Use While Traveling

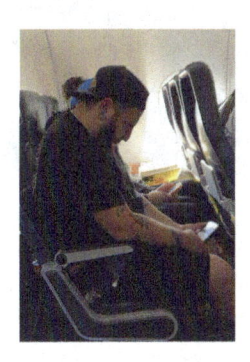

Traveling often means spending more time on devices. Whether you're scrolling through your phone at the gate, working on a laptop in-flight, watching a movie on an iPad, or reading on a tablet during a layover, chances are that you're spending hours in front of a screen. How you use these devices can have a profound impact on your posture and overall comfort.

Think back to the **Candy Cane Theory**…

Every degree your head tilts forward increases the strain on your neck, just like the pressure builds on a bending candy cane. The higher you hold your device, the less strain you place on your neck and shoulders.

Next time you're at the airport, take a moment to look around. Almost everyone is glued to their devices, their heads bent forward to the extreme. On a recent flight, I couldn't help but notice the people sitting across from me. From the moment we boarded, they were hunched over their phones in the classic "candy cane" position. When we landed three hours later, they were still in the exact same posture, their necks and shoulders locked into place.

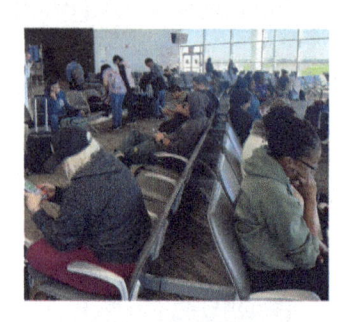

The thing is, they won't feel the effects immediately. Give it a day or two—maybe three—and they'll start wondering why their necks or shoulders suddenly start aching. They might even blame it on an old injury or convince themselves it's serious enough to consider injections or surgery.

The solution is simple: every degree higher you hold your device matters.

Tools like a portable laptop stand are must-haves for maintaining good posture while traveling. Whether you're on a plane, waiting at the terminal, or working in a hotel room, staying mindful of your posture can prevent those delayed, seemingly "mystery" aches and pains. Look up, adjust your position, and invest in your well-being—your future self will thank you.

The Flight Attendant's Challenge

It started with a conversation at the airport. I was waiting to board my flight when I struck up a chat with a flight attendant pulling his suitcase effortlessly through the terminal. As we talked, he mentioned a common issue among his colleagues: shoulder pain.

"Most of us deal with it at some point," he said, adjusting the strap of his bag. "We're taught to pull our suitcases with our palms facing backward, it's supposed to make maneuvering easier. But after years of doing that, it starts to wear on you."

His words struck a chord. I'd seen this issue with flight attendants and with everyday travelers. People hauling heavy bags on one shoulder or dragging suitcases behind them without a second thought.

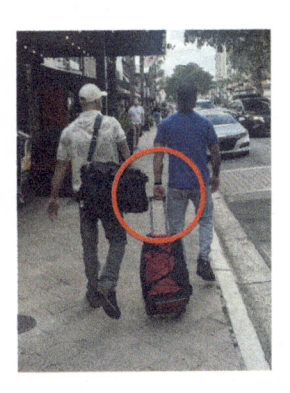

I explained how pulling a suitcase with the palm facing backward could lead to shoulder impingement over time. This posture forces the shoulder into an unnatural position, especially during long hauls through sprawling airports.

"It's like carrying a heavy purse on one shoulder," I told him. "It creates imbalanced loading, which can lead to discomfort or even chronic pain."

His eyes lit up as I shared a simple solution. Switch to pulling the suitcase with the palms facing forward, switch arms often, or opt for a four-wheeled suitcase to allow for more natural movement options, such as holding it in a "bicep curl" position. . By engaging the biceps and keeping the shoulder neutral, the strain is significantly reduced.

A week later, he reached out to me. "I tried your suggestion," he wrote. "It felt strange at first, but my shoulder already feels better. I even shared it with my crew, and they couldn't believe the difference such a small change made!"

This isn't just for flight attendants. Everyday travelers carrying bags on one shoulder or dragging suitcases the same way for hours can experience the same issues. A quick switch in technique—*alternating shoulders, engaging the core, or adjusting your grip*—can prevent imbalances, ensure a pain-free journey, and keep you from returning home with more than just jet lag.

Chapter 6
Shoulder Secrets

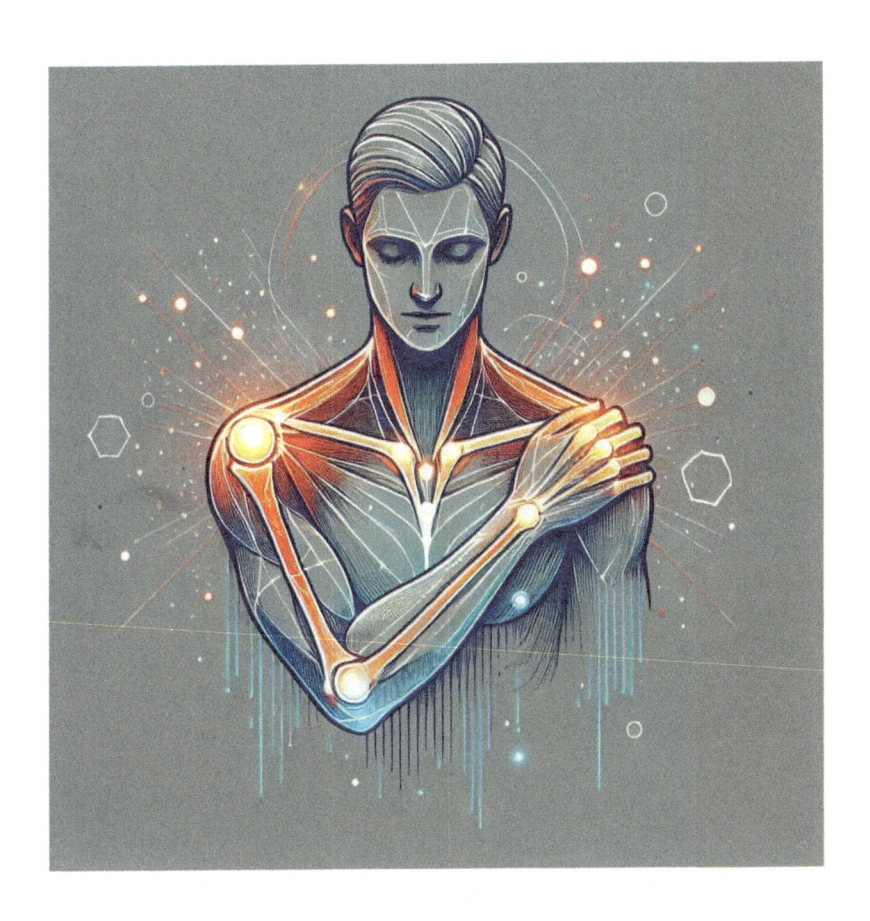

Shoulder Secrets

Why Does My Shoulder Hurt, and What's Really Going On?

Let's start with a profound truth that might surprise you: roughly half of all shoulder pain isn't from injury or age—it's from how we unconsciously move through our daily lives. By using the Slight Motion Method we've discovered that most people are unknowingly performing, what we call "self-impingement", dozens of times each day.

Do You Have Shoulder Pain? Could It Be Impingement?

If you're struggling with shoulder pain, one of the most common culprits is **shoulder impingement**. More than half of all shoulder pain is due to shoulder impingement. But what exactly is impingement, and why does it happen? Shoulder impingement occurs when the tendons or bursa in the shoulder become pinched during arm movements, particularly if you have **forward or rounded shoulders**.

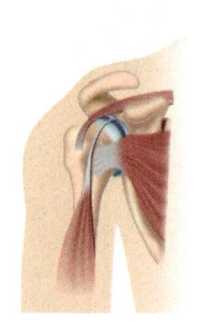

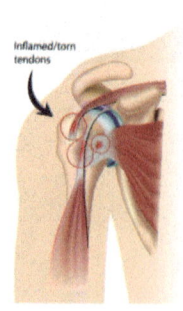

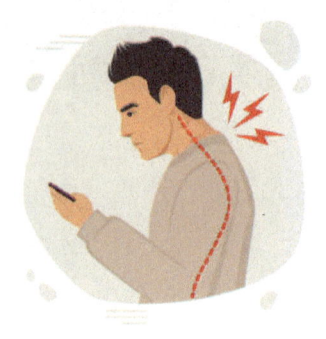

This is where the **Slight Motion Method** can help identify subtle postural imbalances and faulty movement patterns that can lead to impingement. The key to healing shoulder pain is understanding the mechanics of your shoulder and recognizing the activities that might be causing it. With expert guidance from a **Slight Motion Specialist**, we can identify subtle habits that may have gone unnoticed, yet are key contributors to your pain.

What Is This "Rotator Cuff" Everyone Talks About?

You've heard the term, but did you know the rotator cuff isn't just one thing? It's actually a sophisticated system of four muscles working together like a perfectly orchestrated symphony. When one musician plays out of tune—or in our case, when one muscle isn't working properly—the entire performance suffers.

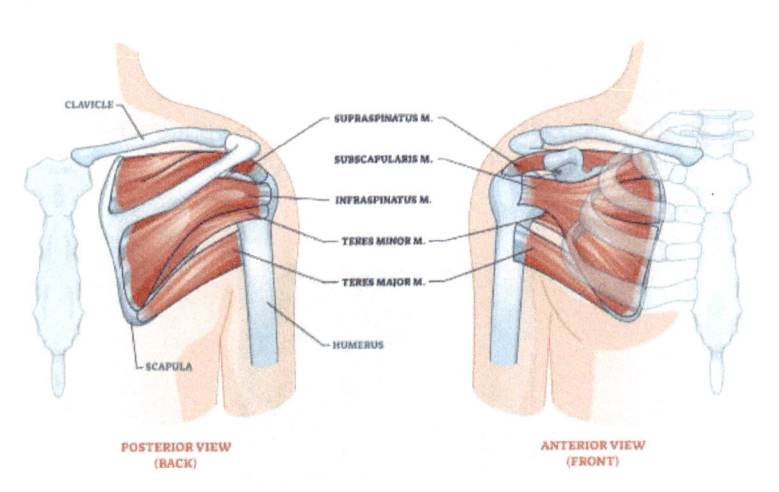

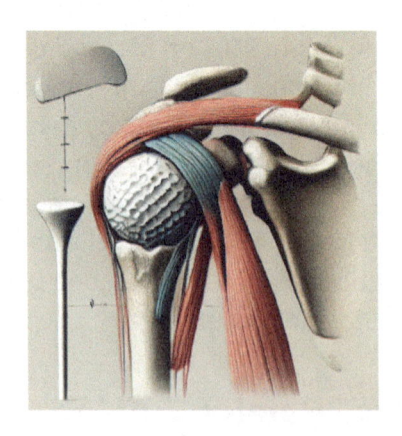

Your shoulder is a ball-and-socket joint. Think of how a golf ball sits on a tee. The rotator cuff muscles are like four fingers holding that ball perfectly centered in place, allowing the shoulder to move smoothly in any direction. When these muscles aren't working properly, the "golf ball" starts rubbing against the "tee," creating what we call impingement.

Look around in any coffee shop, office, or red light. What do you see? People hunched over phones, rounded shoulders, heads forward. This position isn't just uncomfortable—it's literally squeezing the space where your rotator cuff needs to move, like trying to dance in a crowded elevator.

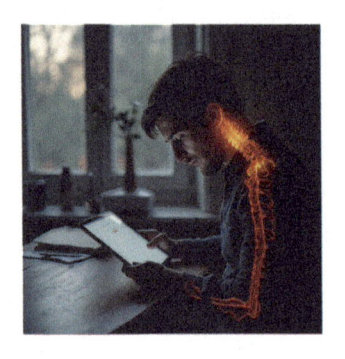

Here's a quick breakdown:

- **Supraspinatus**: The most commonly involved and injured muscle with impingement, especially in the subacromial space. It functions to assist the deltoid muscle in lifting the arm out to the side. Its tendon travels under the acromion and gets compressed due to faulty mechanics in the shoulder. The bone basically becomes a saw to this tendon, which is why it's the most commonly torn rotator cuff muscle.
- **Infraspinatus:** Helps with external rotation of the shoulder and prevents dislocation or excessive movement during arm and shoulder activities.
    - Examples of Activities Using the Infraspinatus
        - Throwing a ball
        - Reaching behind your body
        - Rotating your arm outward, such as turning a doorknob or swinging a racket
- **Teres Minor:** Also helps with external rotation and helps bring the arm closer to the body
- **Subscapularis:** Primary muscle responsible for internal rotation of the shoulder and assists in pulling the arm closer to the body
    - Examples of Activities Using the Subscapularis
        - Reaching behind your back (e.g., tucking in a shirt).
        - Turning your arm inward, such as rotating a steering wheel.
        - Performing movements that require inward pulling or pushing.

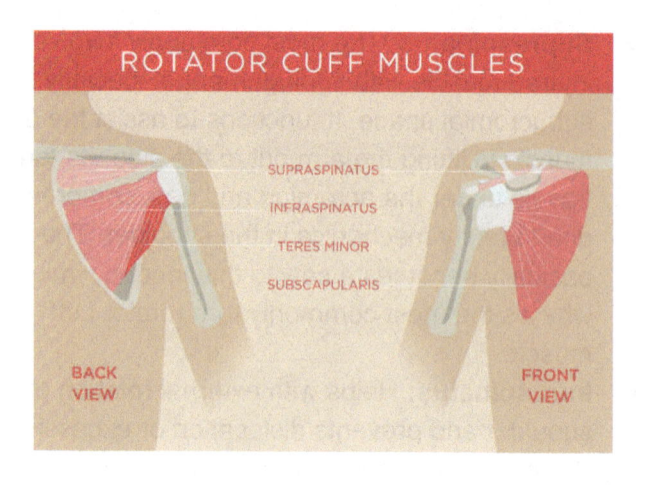

ROTATOR CUFF MUSCLES

SUPRASPINATUS
INFRASPINATUS
TERES MINOR
SUBSCAPULARIS

BACK VIEW

FRONT VIEW

Do you spend a lot of time sitting at a desk, using your phone, or driving? If so, these postures affect a lot more than just your neck and spine. Chances are your shoulders are also rounded forward, which can significantly increase your risk of impingement. When you try to lift your arm in this position, the space in your shoulder joint narrows, pinching the rotator cuff tendons causing inflammation and pain.

The Modern Posture Predicament

Imagine your shoulder joint is like a revolving door in a busy hotel. When you stand tall with good posture, that door spins smoothly, letting people (or in our case, tendons and muscles) pass through effortlessly. But what happens when you're hunched over your phone or laptop? It's like someone has tilted that revolving door forward. Now everyone has to squeeze through at an awkward angle, creating friction, jamming the mechanism, and eventually causing damage.

This is exactly what's happening in your shoulder when you maintain that forward-rounded posture. Your supraspinatus tendon is forced to slide through a now-narrowed space every time you lift your arm; like a person trying to squeeze through that tilted revolving door. Do this hundreds of times a day while texting, typing, or scrolling, and it's no wonder your shoulder starts complaining!

Are Your Daily Activities Making Your Shoulder Pain Worse?

Some everyday activities can worsen shoulder pain and increase the likelihood of impingement:

- **Do you reach across your body to open doors or grab things?** This cross-body motion compresses the shoulder joint and can cause pain. Try not to open sliding glass doors with your opposite arm, having to reach across your body and pull.
- **Do you reach into the back seat while driving?** The twisting, cross-body motion required for this action puts a lot of stress on the shoulder joint and can lead to impingement or rotator cuff injury over time.

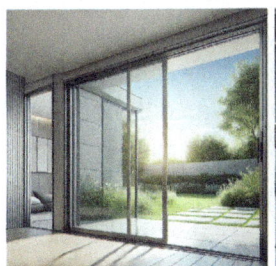

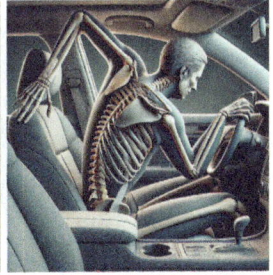

The Sliding Door Revelation

I had a client who came to me with persistent shoulder pain that was starting to limit her recreational activities. She couldn't figure out what was causing it, or why it wasn't getting better despite rest and therapy.

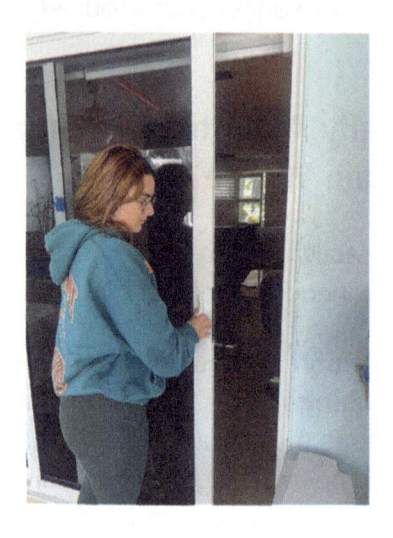

One day, I visited her house to get a better sense of her daily movements. As we talked, she casually got up to let her dog out through a sliding glass door. That's when it all clicked.

The door slid from right to left, and every time she opened it, she used her right arm, extending it awkwardly and pulling at an angle that mimicked the shoulder impingement test. She did this multiple times a day since her dog was particularly active. Was it the cause of the initial injury? Probably not. Was it a contributing factor to why her shoulder wasn't getting better as quickly as it could? Absolutely. This small, repetitive motion was perpetuating the irritation cycle and keeping her pain alive.

We discussed it right then and there. I showed her how to use her left arm instead, keeping the movement closer to her body, almost like a bicep curl. The difference was immediate. She could feel how this adjustment stopped irritating her shoulder and broke the cycle that had been preventing her recovery.

The lesson here? Be mindful of how you open doors—or perform any repetitive motion. Sometimes, it's the smallest, most routine actions that perpetuate pain. Try to avoid activities or habits that mimic this shoulder impingement and keep your movements intentional and safe. Even something as simple as switching arms can make all the difference.

The Car Alignment Analogy

Your shoulder is like a car's wheel alignment. When everything's properly aligned, you can drive smoothly without wearing out your tires. But if your alignment is off (like with rounded shoulders), every mile you drive creates uneven wear and tear. You might not notice it immediately, but over time, that misalignment causes premature degeneration. Similarly, poor shoulder positioning doesn't hurt right away, but repeatedly lifting your arm in that misaligned state gradually damages the tissues.

The Bartender's Shoulder

I worked with a bartender named Scarlett, who'd been in the industry for over a decade. She came to me frustrated and in pain. "It's my shoulder," she said, rolling it gingerly. "I can't even lift it some days, and I don't know why. It's not like I'm lifting heavy stuff—it's just bottles and glasses."

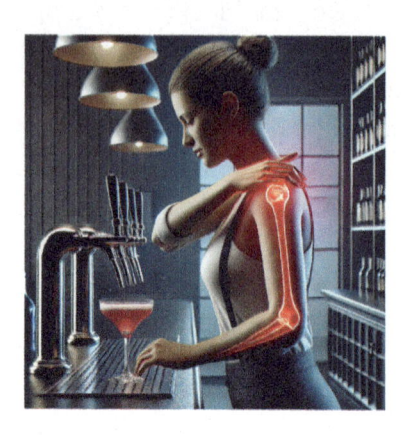

Scarlett's story wasn't unique. Over the years, I've seen countless bartenders dealing with similar issues. Their pain wasn't coming from the weight of the bottles, but from how they poured drinks. I asked Scarlett to show me how she worked behind the bar, and within seconds, the issue became clear.

Every time Scarlett poured a drink, she reached to the side, angling her shoulder in a way that mimicked the test we use to diagnose shoulder impingement or a rotator cuff tear. By keeping the glass off to the side, she was essentially self-impinging her shoulder dozens, if not hundreds, of times a shift. Add in the repetitive motions of scooping ice, shaking cocktails, and grabbing bottles, and it was no wonder her shoulder was crying out for relief.

The solution was simple but effective. I told Scarlett, "Next time you pour, move the glass closer to your dominant side—the same side you're pouring with." By bringing the motion to the center of her body, she could pour without twisting or overloading her shoulder. We also worked on building ambidexterity, encouraging her to use both arms for tasks behind the bar to distribute the workload more evenly.

A few weeks later, Scarlett came back with a grin. "I'm not saying I'm 100% pain-free yet," she said, "but it's already so much better. I didn't realize such a small change could make such a big difference."

Since then, I've shared this advice with other bartenders, and the results have been consistent. By moving the glass to the center or closer to the pouring arm, they reduce the strain on their shoulders and prevent further impingement. Some even find their shifts less exhausting as they adopt a more balanced approach to their movements.

Next time you're at a bar, think about the mechanics behind the drink you're being served. How is the bartender pouring? Are they scooping ice repeatedly or shaking cocktails with one arm? These small habits, when adjusted, can mean the difference between chronic pain and a thriving career. For bartenders like Scarlett, the fix was as simple as shifting a glass—and it's made all the difference.

The Power of Switching Sides

Do you brush your teeth? Of course you do, it's something you do every single day. But here's the question: why not use that time to get better, not just at brushing, but at unlocking the full potential of your body?

I was a good soccer player on one of the top teams in the nation, I wanted to push myself to the next level. My left foot was solid, I trained it every day, but it wasn't great. While on a team competing at the highest level, good wasn't enough. I needed my left foot to be as precise and accurate as my right.

That's when I started brushing my teeth with my non-dominant hand. It seemed small, but the results were huge. By training a whole different part of my brain, I rewired how I moved and gained better control over my left side. Slowly, that coordination transferred to the field. My left foot went from good to great.

I didn't keep it to myself, either. I told my teammates, "Start brushing your teeth with your other hand!" At first, they laughed, but when they saw the improvement in my game, they joined in. Over time, we all became more precise and confident with our non-dominant legs, and that edge took us even further. We went on to win three state titles.

How does this apply to you? We have two arms and two legs, but most of us rely far too much on one side. Training your non-dominant side isn't just about better coordination, it's about creating new neural pathways that make everyday tasks safer and more efficient.

Imagine you're reaching for something on the left side of your body with your right hand. That cross-body motion compresses your shoulder and can lead to unnecessary strain. If you've trained your left side, your body can respond naturally, keeping you safer and moving smarter.

I've seen this principle work off the field too. A college teammate who worked as a server became faster and more efficient at dealing with checks and tasks by training her non-dominant hand. A bartender I worked with learned to pour drinks, scoop ice, and grab bottles with both hands, reducing the strain from constant cross-body reaching.

The beauty of this practice is its simplicity. Start with something you already do, like brushing your teeth. It might feel awkward at first, but stick with it. Over time, you'll gain better control of your movements, protect your spine, and unlock a whole new level of coordination.

For me and my teammates, it led to championships. For you, it might mean moving through life with more ease, safety, and efficiency. So, next time you pick up your toothbrush, ask yourself: which hand are you using? It's time to do better.

The Case of the Housekeeper's Shoulder

One day, my housekeeper walked in with an elbow brace. Naturally, I asked, "What's going on with your arm?" He explained that he'd been dealing with shoulder pain ever since cleaning windows a few weeks ago.

As we talked, I asked about his habits. Did he use his phone often? "Not really," he replied, which seemed like the end of that line of questioning. But something wasn't adding up.

I decided to dig a little deeper. "What about before bed? Do you use your phone then?" His face lit up as he admitted, "Oh yeah, I play this game on my phone for about an hour before I sleep." Curious, I asked him to describe how he set himself up.

"Well," he said, "I prop myself up with a few pillows and rest the phone on my chest while I play."

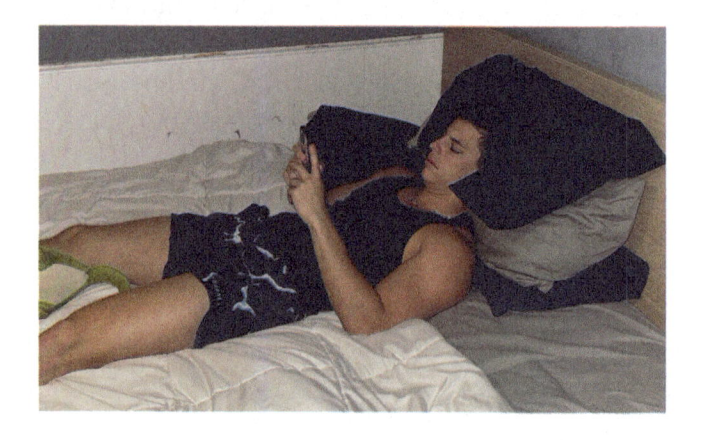

And that's when it all clicked. His so-called shoulder pain wasn't from cleaning windows—it was radiculopathy stemming from his spine. The combination of multiple pillows and the awkward angle of his neck while playing his game was putting pressure on his cervical spine, irritating the nerves that traveled down his arm.

I explained what was happening and suggested he adjust his setup. By supporting his head properly and holding the phone at a neutral angle, he could reduce the strain on his neck and stop the nerve irritation.

The takeaway? Sometimes, what seems like one issue—like shoulder pain—is actually something entirely different. By looking beyond the obvious and understanding daily habits, we can uncover the real causes of pain and address them effectively. It's a reminder to be mindful of how we position our bodies, even during something as simple as unwinding with a game before bed.

The Case of the Hands Behind the Back

When I was still seeing clients in the clinic, I worked with a woman who had persistent shoulder pain. Her recovery was frustrating, she'd get better for a while, then her pain would return without any clear reason. She was very active and loved walking, so we chalked it up to her busy lifestyle.

One day, by chance, I saw her walking down the street. That's when everything clicked. As she strolled, her arms were clasped behind her back—a habit that seemed harmless at first glance. But to me, it was a clear problem: she was unknowingly impinging her own shoulder.

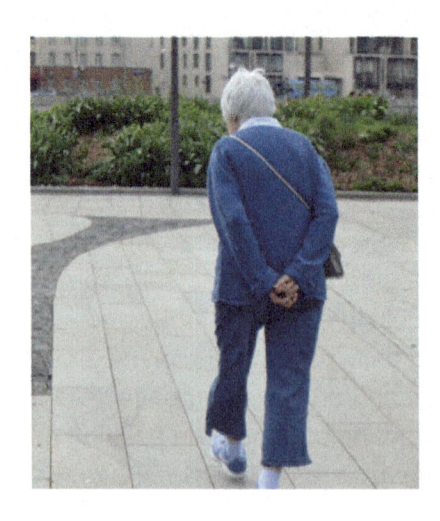

At her next session, I brought it up. "Do you usually walk with your arms behind your back?" I asked. She nodded, surprised that I'd noticed. I explained how this position could compress her shoulder joint, exacerbating her pain.

We worked on changing this habit, and she significantly reduced the time she spent walking in that posture. Within weeks, her pain was gone for good.

Another client came to me with a similar issue. She mentioned that someone had once told her to hold her arms behind her back while standing to help her "stand up straighter." She had adopted this position as a default, thinking it was good for her posture. I quickly explained that while it might feel like it's helping her stand tall, it was actually causing unnecessary strain on her shoulders and perpetuating her pain.

The takeaway? Be mindful of how you position your arms, whether you're walking, standing, or simply chatting with friends.

Holding your arms behind your back might seem like a harmless—or even helpful—habit, but it can do more harm than good, especially for your shoulders. If you're trying to improve your posture, there are far better ways to do it than risking impingement and discomfort.

Sometimes, recovery isn't about big changes; it's about noticing the small, everyday habits that might be holding you back. For these clients, letting go of the "hands behind the back" posture was the key to moving forward pain-free.

Palms Up, Thumbs Up: A Core Principle

One of the core principles I teach my clients is simple but incredibly effective: palms up, thumbs up.

When sitting, try resting your palms facing up. This position, often used in yoga, naturally opens your chest, relaxes your shoulders, and promotes a balanced, upright posture. Don't believe me? Give it a try. Place your palms up and notice how your body feels—open, upright, and free. Now turn your palms down. Instantly, your body rolls forward and closes in, creating tension and restriction.

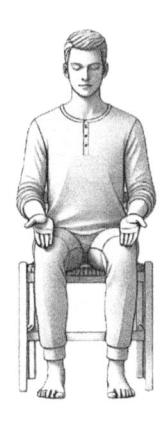

This principle applies to walking, too. We don't want to move through life with our palms down, like a meathead with puffed-up shoulders and a closed-off chest. Instead, aim to walk with your hands in a neutral, thumbs-forward position—what I jokingly call the "karate chop" stance. This small adjustment keeps your chest open, improves your posture, and reduces strain on your shoulders.

It's a habit that extends beyond posture; it's about being intentional with your body's positioning. Most of the things I teach are small, actionable changes you can implement at home or in your daily routine. Life is about controlling the controllables, and this is one you can practice every day.

Sometimes, my clients like to have a little fun with it. Whenever I visit bars where I've treated bartenders, they'll walk up to me with their palms open and big grins on their faces, just to mess with me—because it looks funny. But what's amazing is how much the lesson sticks. They've become more aware of their posture, and it's clear they're carrying themselves differently now.

Whether you're sitting, walking, or simply standing in line, remember: palms up, thumbs up. It's a small shift with a big impact, and your body will thank you for it.

I had a client who recently started walking to the gym and developed neck and shoulder pain. Turns out it was because he would carry a heavy gym bag on only one side of his shoulder.

A solution: turn this into a suitcase carry to balance out the weight and take off pressure from the shoulder.

Upper Body Exercise...Are You Doing More Harm Than Good?

For people who work out and have shoulder pain, I can usually guess some of the exercises they're doing. As soon as they're aware of it and make the necessary modifications, their pain goes away.

Many common shoulder exercises actually create impingement. Let's reconsider:
- Lateral raise to 90 degrees
    - Try to modify the range to 45 degrees instead
- Traditional overhead press
    - Try lifting slightly anterior instead of directly overhead
- Overhead triceps extension
    - Try tricep extension on cables instead

Rethinking Shoulder Workouts: Train Smarter, Not Harder

As the name suggests, the rotator cuff plays a crucial role in rotational movements and stabilizing the shoulder joint. Unlike larger shoulder muscles that generate power, the rotator cuff's primary job is stability and keeping the ball of the humerus centered in the socket. Internal and external rotation are the primary muscle actions of the rotator cuff. Weaknesses or imbalances in these small, but essential muscles can lead to pain or injury when performing traditional lifting or overhead exercises. Incorporating targeted rotator cuff exercises into your upper body workout routine will improve joint mechanics, reduce injury risk, and enhance overall shoulder function.

Below, are some rotator cuff exercises you should incorporate into your routine:

- **Internal Rotation & Progressions**
    - Internal rotation engages the **subscapularis** muscle, supporting functional movements like reaching and lifting

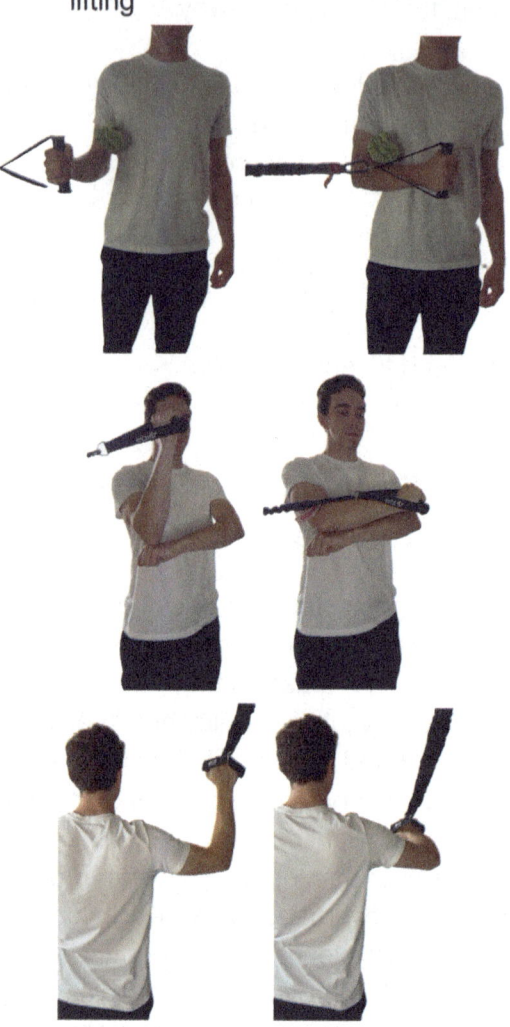

- **External Rotation & Progressions**
    - External rotation targets the **infraspinatus** and **teres minor** muscles, improving stabilization of the shoulder joint

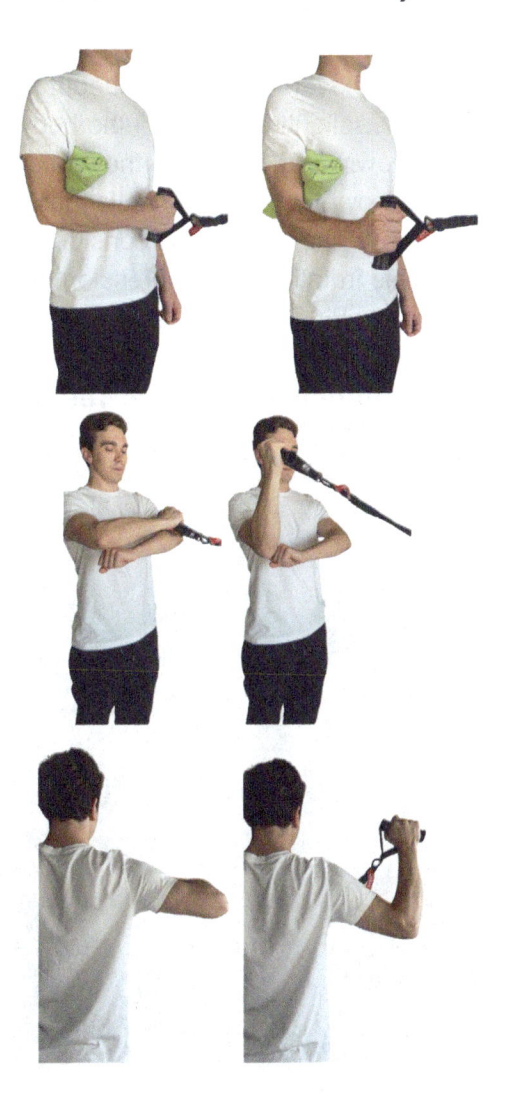

Thumbs Up 👍 Vs. Thumbs Down 👎

When assessing shoulder impingement or potential rotator cuff involvement, one of the key diagnostic tests we use is the *Empty Can Test*. This special test is performed by having the person elevate their arm to about 90 degrees in the scapular plane (slightly forward of the body), with the thumb pointing downward, similar to the motion of emptying a can. Downward resistance is then applied. If this position causes pain, the test is considered positive, indicating possible irritation or compression of the rotator cuff tendons, particularly the supraspinatus.

Impingement Special Tests

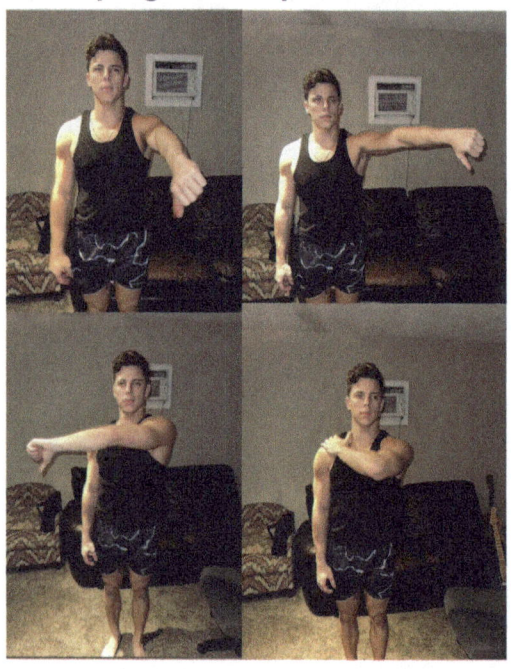

While this position is useful for diagnostic purposes, it's not ideal for exercise or strength training. When you perform movements with your thumbs pointed down, especially under load, you're repeatedly placing the shoulder in a mechanically vulnerable position. This can lead to cumulative stress, inflammation, and over time, contribute to tendon degeneration or impingement-related injuries.

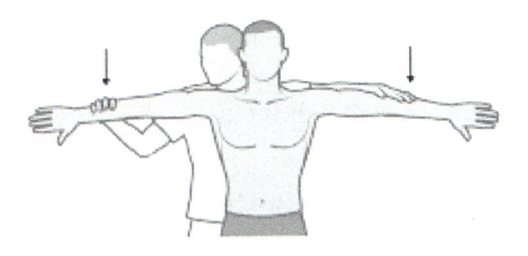

We encourage the 👍THUMBS UP 👍 position when doing forward or lateral raises to maintain improved mechanics on the shoulder joint, especially when loading with weight. "Thumbs up position" promotes external rotation of the shoulder, which helps maintain a more open subacromial space, reduces unnecessary stress on the rotator cuff, and supports healthier shoulder mechanics.

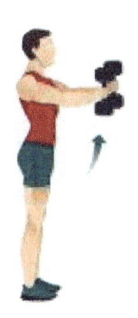

Most everyday movements naturally happen with a thumb-up position, like lifting a gallon of milk into the fridge. Now, imagine trying to lift that same gallon with your palm facing down—it would feel awkward and put more strain on your shoulder. This is the same position many people use when doing front raises at the gym. While it does target the front of your shoulder more (anterior deltoid), it can also worsen shoulder pain or impingement if you're already experiencing discomfort. The key to shoulder health is about moving it in ways that work with your body, not against its functional movements.

Key Takeaway For Lasting Shoulder Health

Shoulder health isn't just about what you do in the gym, it's about how you move all day, every day. The way you lift, reach, and carry things matters just as much as the exercises you perform. By becoming more aware of your movement patterns, making strategic adjustments, and respecting your shoulder's natural biomechanics, you can prevent pain before it starts. True strength comes not just from muscle, but from mindful movement. Balance is key. Using both sides of your body equally helps prevent overuse and muscular imbalances that can lead to pain. When you understand the mind-body connection, you move with intention, ensuring every motion supports, not strains, your joints. Your shoulders are built for longevity; when you treat them right, they'll support you for a lifetime.

Chapter 7
Thoracic Thoughts

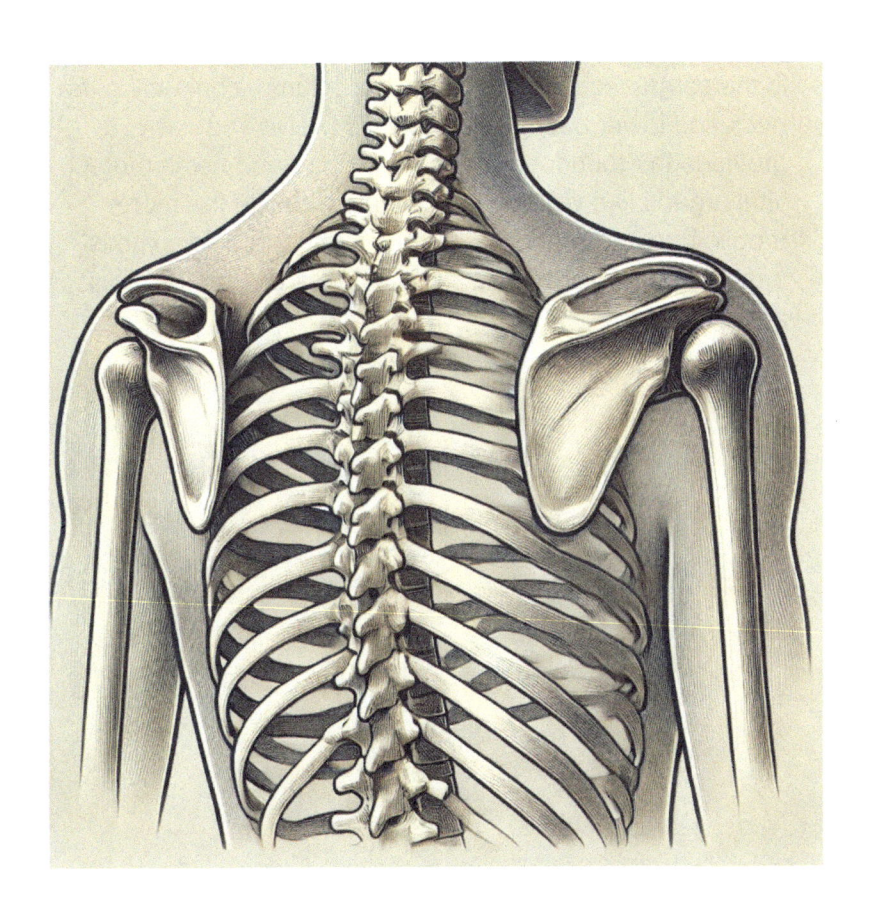

Thoracic Thoughts

What is the Thoracic Spine?

The thoracic spine, often overlooked but vitally important, is the central section of your spinal column, connecting the neck and lower back. Comprised of twelve vertebrae, it provides the foundation for your ribcage and helps protect vital organs like your heart and lungs. Unlike the more mobile cervical and lumbar regions, the thoracic spine is designed for stability, offering a balance between support and flexibility.

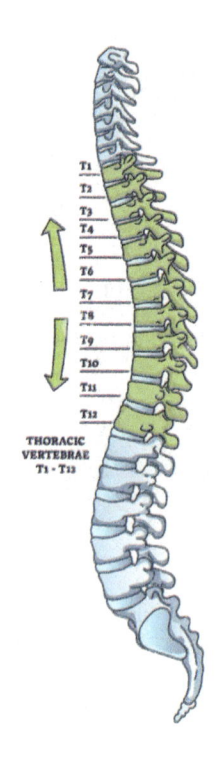

However, this balance can be a double-edged sword. The thoracic spine is frequently the unsung culprit behind back and mid-back pain. Its relatively rigid structure, combined with poor posture habits like slouching or prolonged sitting, places immense strain on this area. Over time, this strain can lead to stiffness, discomfort, and even nerve irritation. Understanding the thoracic spine and its role in your body is the first step toward addressing and alleviating mid-back pain.

Do You Twist Your Spine First Thing In the Morning?

Miles came to me with persistent mid-back pain that just wouldn't quit after moving to a new apartment. After one session, he felt amazing—pain-free for the first time in months. But within days, his discomfort came roaring back. This back-and-forth puzzled us both, so I started digging into his daily routine

When I visited his apartment, I noticed a few big boxes in the living room. "What's in those?" I asked. He shrugged and said, "Oh, those are the new bedside tables. My wife didn't like them, so she's planning to get different ones."

That was my lightbulb moment. Our spine is fragile in the morning especially after hours in one position. Without bedside tables, Miles had developed a peculiar habit: every morning and night, he twisted his torso and strained his mid-back reaching down to the floor to grab his phone. "It's such a small thing," he said, "I can't believe it could matter."

But those small, repeated movements are often the root of chronic pain. "Think of your spine as a delicate suspension bridge," I explained. "Every time you contort it to grab something, you create tiny stresses. Over time, those stresses add up, leaving you with pain that feels like it came out of nowhere."

We made one simple change: while waiting for new tables, Miles placed a small stool next to his bed to keep his phone within easy reach. The result? His pain disappeared—and this time, it stayed gone. It wasn't a complicated fix, but it made all the difference.

This experience got me thinking about how many other habits might contribute to similar pain. For instance, do you eat at a proper table, or are you hunching over a coffee table, couch, or low surface? Miles also mentioned he sometimes experienced pain while eating, which brought to mind an old etiquette lesson: always bring your soup to you, not the other way around. Even dog bowls are now often elevated to spare pets' necks and spines—if it's important for animals, shouldn't it be just as important for us?

Do You Pull Items From Your Back Seat?

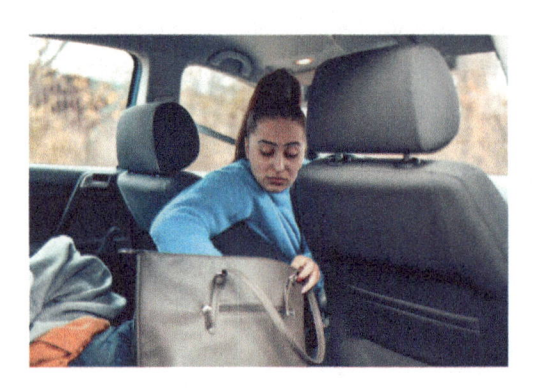

Do you ever put items in your back seat and pull them to the front? It's a habit that seems harmless but can easily lead to pulling a muscle or even slipping a disc. I've had several clients who reported severe back pain after twisting awkwardly to grab something from their car's back seat. Are you mindful of how you move when retrieving items from your car? That one small motion could be the cause of your thoracic pain.

The Door Saga: Unveiling the Unexpected

Pain often hides in the most unexpected places, and sometimes the root cause isn't what we think. Mia came to us with severe mid-thoracic and rib pain. Doctors had labeled it a "slipped rib," a diagnosis that left her frustrated and searching for answers. Together, we explored her daily habits, from her posture to her workspace ergonomics. Nothing stood out as the smoking gun—at least not initially.

But the truth was waiting just outside her door.

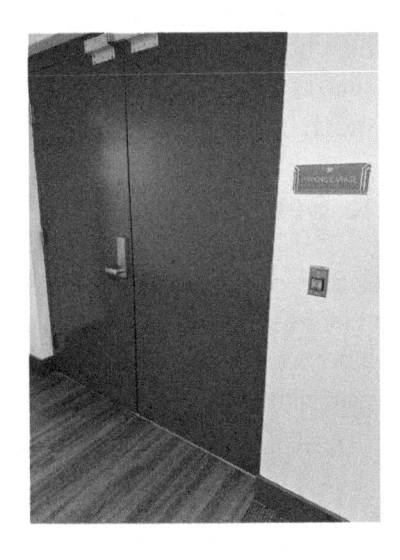

After a session, I headed to my car, only to be momentarily stumped by the mechanics of her apartment door. It was a two-door exit: you pressed a button on the right, but had to simultaneously reach across to open the left door. That awkward twist—pressing on the right and pulling on the left—was subtle but insidious. It was a movement she repeated multiple times daily without even thinking about it, often while carrying a load—whether it was a backpack, a purse, or even a bag of trash. The added weight amplified the strain on her thoracic spine and rib cage, making the seemingly minor habit even more damaging.

I couldn't shake the realization. That repetitive, asymmetric motion—reaching and twisting—was creating the perfect storm for her rib pain. The muscles and joints in her thoracic region were under constant strain, leading to her symptoms.

Once I brought this to Mia's attention, the pieces clicked into place. We worked together to modify how she interacted with the door, exploring ways to minimize the twist. Within weeks, her pain began to subside. She was floored by how such a small detail in her environment could cause so much discomfort.

Is Making the Bed Hurting Your Back?

Claire's mid-back pain had her at her wit's end. A mother of three and the family host, she couldn't figure out why her back had started bothering her. "It started right after we had guests," she admitted.

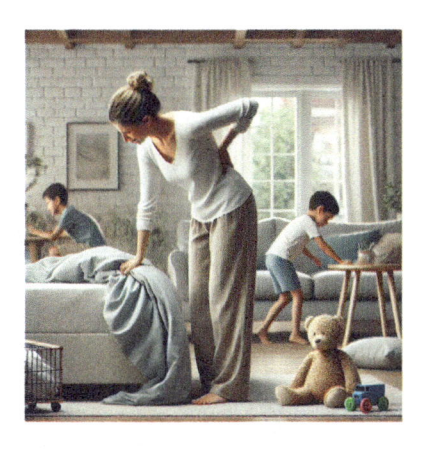

That was the clue I needed. Claire had spent days setting up and taking down beds for her visitors. Bending, tucking, and lifting—small movements repeated over and over. Then, there was her time with the grandkids, crawling on the floor and picking them up. Her core wasn't ready for the strain, and her mid-back was bearing the brunt.

We focused on strengthening her core and adjusting her movements. For example, she started becoming more aware of her spine twisting movements and remembered to modify along the way. Within weeks, Claire was pain-free and back to entertaining—without sacrificing her back in the process.

Is Folding Laundry Causing Your Pain?

Another client, Megan, had similar mid-back discomfort. She was baffled—it didn't seem like she was doing anything strenuous. But when we talked through her daily habits, one activity stood out: folding clothes. She always folded her laundry on her bed, and her bed was low, which meant she was constantly bending over at an awkward, low angle.

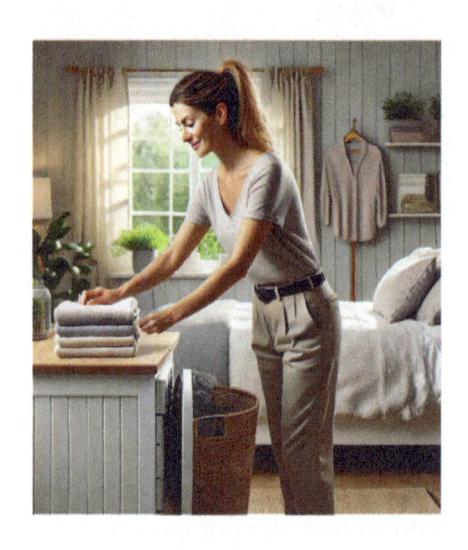

I suggested a small adjustment: move the task to a dresser or countertop, where she wouldn't have to hunch. Combined with mindfulness about her posture and regular stretching, this simple change eased her discomfort significantly. "I never thought something as mundane as laundry could be the culprit," she said, "but now my back feels so much better."

Still, Megan had her own solution ready. "Honestly, maybe I just shouldn't fold laundry at all," she joked, "Wrinkled clothes are in, right?" We both laughed, but she quickly admitted her back felt much better after making the small change. "Turns out laundry and I can still get along—just at a more spine-friendly height."

How high is your washer and dryer?

Do You Reach for Things From High Shelves?

How often do you reach for dishes on high shelves or put them really high up in cabinets? If you consistently overreach with one side of your body, especially if you're right-side dominant, this repetitive motion can put unnecessary strain on your thoracic spine. I've worked with clients who habitually reach across their body with one arm, twisting their body to grab items, leading to muscle imbalances and, over time, persistent pain. Have you noticed a tendency to favor one side when lifting or reaching? It might be a small habit, but it could be playing a big role in your middle back discomfort.

Do you ever need to reach up high in the shower to adjust the settings or move showerheads? I experienced mid-back pain myself when I had to reach up to switch the lever to use both shower heads. Repeatedly reaching high or awkwardly extending your arms could put strain on your mid-back, causing discomfort. Could simple movements like adjusting your shower settings be contributing to your pain?

Are You a Leaner?

Do you lean to one side when sitting or standing? If so, you could be contributing to scoliosis-like shifts in your spine. While scoliosis is often considered genetic, in my practice, I've found that many people with scoliosis are big "leaners." Their spines don't just shift without reason—repeated leaning or side-lying in awkward positions can create imbalances over time.

For example, some people lie on their side, propping their head up with their arm in a triangle shape or they use more than one pillow. Could this habit be worsening your scoliosis or mid-back pain?

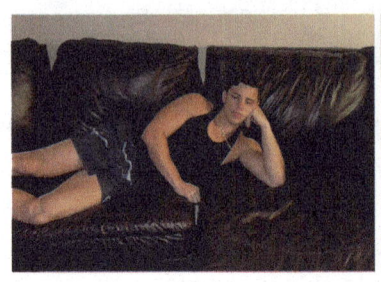

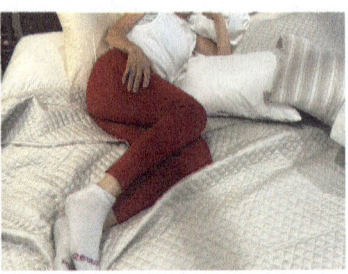

Samantha came to me with persistent mid-back discomfort, which she immediately attributed to her scoliosis. But as we performed a Slight Motion Assessment, another clue became obvious: the armrest on her office chair was visibly worn—on one side. "Do you always lean like that?" I asked, pointing out the uneven wear.

She looked at the armrest, surprised. "I guess I do," she admitted, before adding, "But doesn't scoliosis mean my spine is already curved anyway?"

I smiled and explained, "Your spine might have a natural curve from scoliosis, but leaning constantly reinforces that imbalance and makes things worse. Your spine doesn't just shift for no reason—it responds to how you position it every day."

Samantha realized that her leaning habit was more of a daily choice than an inevitability. We worked on breaking it by alternating arm positions, using better chair support, and improving her overall posture.

After a few weeks, her pain subsided, and her chair got a much-needed break from the constant pressure.

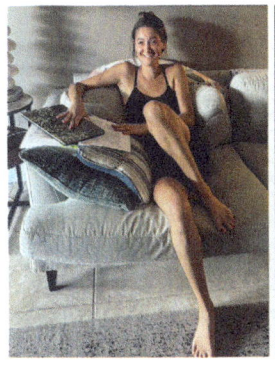

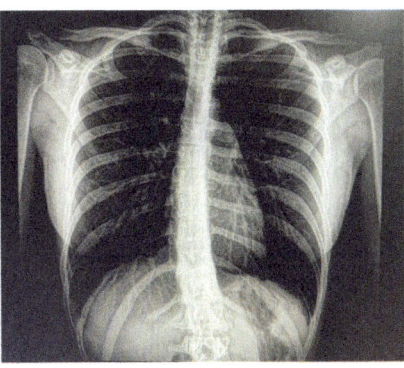

Nearly EVERY client I've treated with scoliosis does the same things.

Scoliosis is often categorized as idiopathic, with no clear cause, or attributed to genetics, where hereditary factors are believed to play a role. Approximately 65% of scoliosis cases are idiopathic, while genetic factors contribute significantly to the risk of developing the condition, accounting for about 38% of the variance.[8]

Additionally in my practice, I've noticed a striking pattern: every client I've treated with scoliosis exhibits the same habits. They favor certain postures, repeatedly leaning, laying on the couch in weird propped up angles, lying on their side with their elbow bent and head supported by their hand, sleeping with multiple pillows under their head or in the wrong places, or repeatedly performing asymmetrical movements. When I ask these clients if their parents had similar habits, they often respond with a knowing "yes," as though the connection is unsurprising.

This makes me wonder: how much of scoliosis is truly genetic, and how much is the result of learned behaviors passed down through generations? Generational habits.

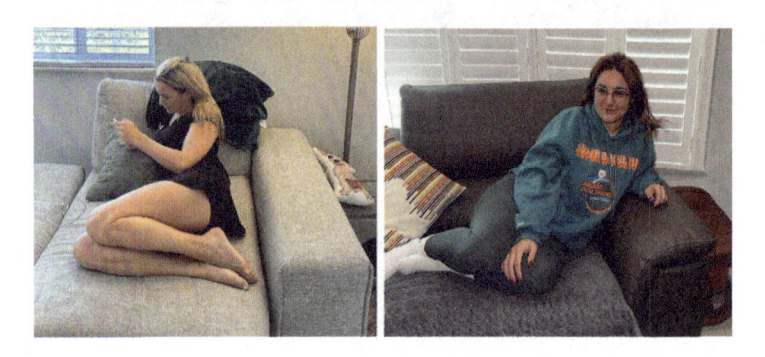

Blaming genetics may seem like the easy way out, but the real story might lie in these shared habits, reinforcing the idea that our daily actions have more impact on our spines than we realize.

Do You Wear the Same Bra On Consecutive Days?

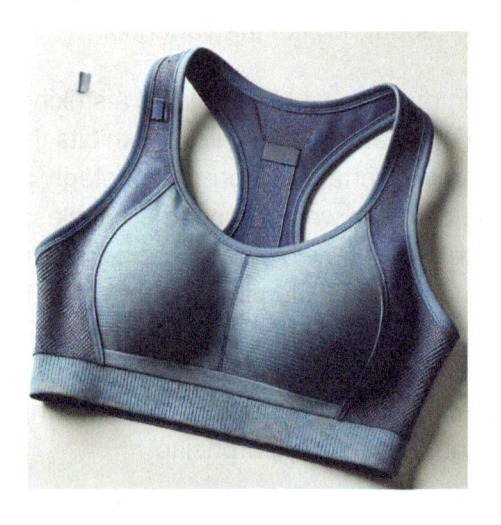

Wearing the same bra repeatedly, especially one with an underwire or clasp hook, can create consistent pressure on the same segment of your thoracic spine.

This is particularly noticeable during activities like sitting or driving, where the bra hook may press directly against your back. Over time, this repeated pressure can lead to discomfort and even slight vertebral shifts. There's even a condition called "bra strap syndrome", where prolonged pressure from tight straps or poorly fitted bras irritates the nerves or tissues beneath them, causing pain and discomfort.

How can you avoid this? Start by checking the fit of your bra. If you notice red marks or indentations on your shoulders, chest, or back when you take it off, it's time to reevaluate. A well-fitting bra should provide support without digging into your body or causing strain. Additionally, rotating your bras regularly can prevent excessive wear and ensure no single area of your spine is subjected to constant pressure.

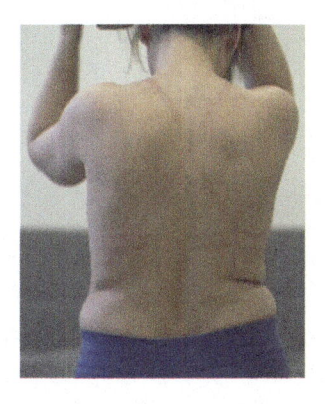

Your bra should support you, not become another source of tension. Paying attention to fit and variety can help reduce unnecessary strain and keep your spine,and you, feeling better.

How Do You Use the Restroom?

Have you ever thought about how your posture while using the restroom could be contributing to your middle back or thoracic pain? One of my clients came to me with significant thoracic pain, and after we ruled out more serious issues, I asked if he had experienced any bowel or bladder changes recently. It turned out he had caught a bug that gave him an upset stomach, and he'd been sitting on the toilet hunched over. After the reset and changing his positioning—sitting more upright—his pain began to subside. Could something as simple as how you sit on the toilet be causing your back pain?

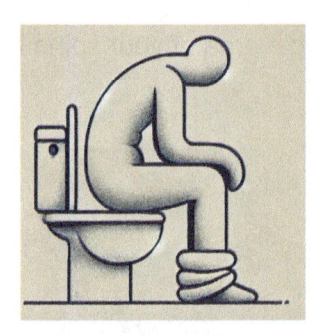

When screening a client with back pain I always ask if any bowel or bladder changes. One time the client mentioned that he caught a stomach bug that some friends had and he was on the toilet more. We realized his seated toilet posture was a contributor to his pain.

Another client reported a possible increase in urination and the rest of his symptoms didn't add up. I suspected his pain might be due to a kidney infection, so I referred him to a physician. Sure enough, it was confirmed it was a kidney infection, not a musculoskeletal issue. This is a powerful reminder that not all back pain is caused by muscle or spine problems; sometimes, the source is something deeper.

Are You Straining on the Toilet?

Men, in particular, tend to sit on the toilet less often than women and might not pay attention to their posture. I've spoken to many male clients who report straining on the toilet, often hunching forward and pushing. This position could be contributing to more than just back pain—it might also increase the risk of hernias. Did you know that hernia prevalence increases as we age, particularly in men? The straining posture can create intra-abdominal pressure, which in turn could push out abdominal organs, leading to a hernia.

Often, hernias develop after a person adopts poor postures, such as hunching over while sitting or straining while using the restroom. If you've had a hernia in the past, or think you may be at risk, it's important to evaluate your posture and habits that could be contributing to your pain.

Studies show that the prevalence of hernias increases with age, particularly in men, with nearly **27% of men over the age of 40** experiencing hernias at some point in their lives.[9]

Hernias occur when there is excessive pressure in the abdominal area, which can push abdominal contents through weakened muscle walls. Maintaining better posture—even on the toilet—can help prevent both thoracic pain and the risk of hernias.

While this issue is more commonly discussed in men, the same poor posture could lead to problems for women, too. Keeping your body in an almost pendulum-like position, where you maintain better alignment, could help prevent pain and other issues. So, how do you sit on the toilet?

How to Relieve Thoracic Pain With Simple Movements

Have You Tried the Open Book Exercise?

Have you ever heard of the "open book" exercise? This simple movement can help relieve thoracic pain by stretching and rotating the muscles in your mid-back. I often recommend doing the open book exercise in the morning to get your body ready for the day's movements, especially if your routine involves a lot of twisting or reaching. It's also a great way to wind down before bed, loosening up any tension that's built up throughout the day. Could adding this simple stretch to your morning or nighttime routine help you find relief from your thoracic pain?

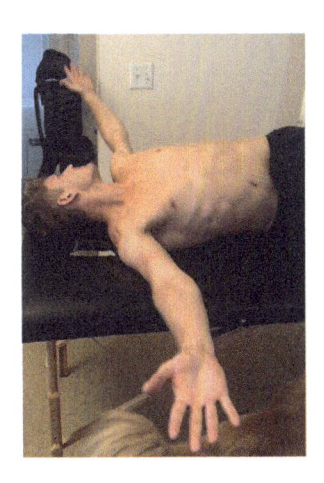

When it comes to thoracic pain, it's often the little things we overlook in our daily lives that add up to big problems. Whether it's how you reach for a bottle, grab something from the back seat, adjust your shower head, or even sit on the toilet, these seemingly insignificant habits can place repeated strain on your body, leading to discomfort and even injury.

The good news? Awareness is the first step to change. By paying attention to these small movements and making thoughtful adjustments, you can not only relieve existing pain but also prevent future issues. From posture tweaks to mindful movement, the path to a healthier, pain-free life often begins with these simple shifts.

Your body works hard for you every day—it's time to work smarter for it. Remember, a little attention to the details of your habits goes a long way toward long-term relief and well-being.

Chapter 8
Lumbar Lessons

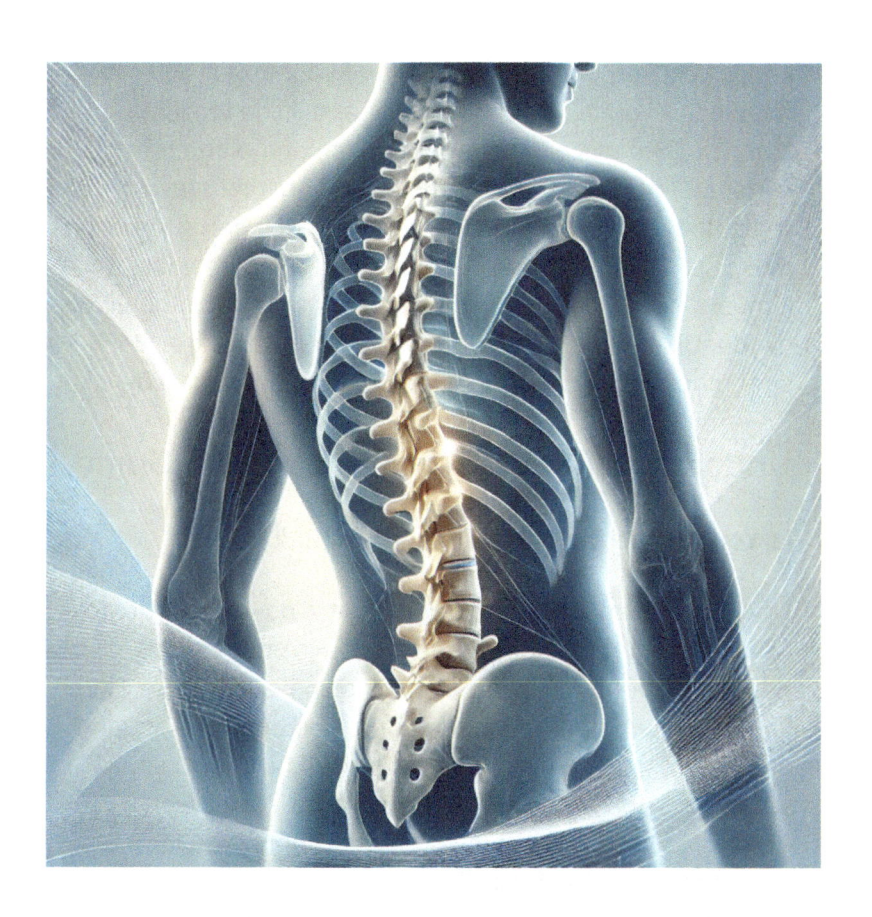

Lumbar Lessons

Your lumbar spine is the workhorse of your back, providing the strength and flexibility needed to support your movements and daily activities. It's the foundation that keeps you upright, bears the load of your upper body, and adapts to everything from bending and lifting to sitting and standing. But this critical region is also one of the most common sources of pain and dysfunction, often falling victim to poor posture, repetitive strain, or weak supporting muscles. In this chapter, we'll explore the mechanics of the lumbar spine, uncover the habits that may be contributing to your discomfort, and share actionable steps to strengthen and protect this essential part of your body.

Understanding the Resilience of the Spine

Is Your Spine Stronger Than You Think?

Do you think your spine is fragile, like a donut filled with jelly? Many people believe their spine is on the verge of breaking, but here's the truth: your spine is more like a tire filled with gum. It is resilient, strong, and built to withstand a lot of pressure. Have you ever said, "I hurt my back 20 years ago, and it's never been the same"? If so, you're not alone. I've heard this from countless clients, and I always smile, knowing that I can probably help them. Did you know that about 80% of adults will experience back pain at some point, but most cases are mechanical, not structural–meaning the problem lies in *how* you move and use your body, not in your spine itself?

Just like we mentioned earlier, we want to think of our spine like a tree. Repeated stress on the same spot weakens it over time, but small shifts in movement give it a chance to adapt and grow stronger. The same principle applies here. Varying your habits is key to keeping your spine resilient. Everything in life that moves, needs to MOVE.

Why Fascia Plays a Key Role in Body-Wide Pain

Your body isn't just a collection of isolated muscles—it's a network of fascia, a web-like connective tissue that links muscles, bones, and organs into a continuous system. Tom Myers' concept of fascial lines explains how tension or dysfunction in one part of the body can travel along these lines, creating pain in seemingly unrelated areas.

In Chapter 3, we discussed how The Superficial Back Line (SBL) runs from your feet, through your hamstrings, along your spine, and up to your skull. If your posture is poor or you have a habit of hunching forward, tension along this line builds, causing neck, back, or hamstring pain. This is called dural tension. That's why chronic back pain isn't always due to disc issues, it could be a fascial imbalance caused by how you move, sit, or sleep.

Can You Balance on One Leg for 30 Seconds?

If not, how do you expect to traverse uneven surfaces or step up confidently without triggering pain? Believe it or not, this seemingly easy 30 second test is proven to be a predictor of life expectancy and risk for falls as you age. Every time you step onto an unknown surface, your body enters "chaos mode," and has to use proprioception to figure out its next move.

Could your lack of balance be contributing to your back pain? Research shows that poor balance is linked to increased risk of chronic back pain, especially in older adults. We've found that a majority of people with low back pain cannot sustain 30 seconds of single leg balance without their legs touching each other. Improving your balance could be the key to alleviating your pain.

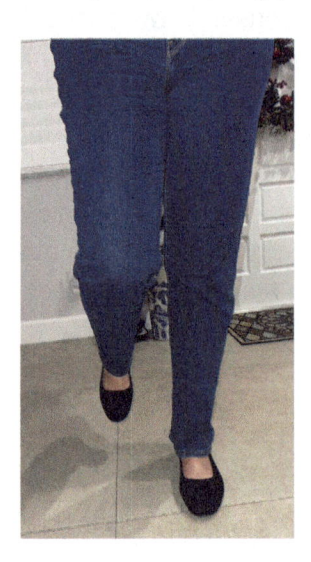

Try this! How many times per day do you have a free 30 seconds? Whether it's waiting for something in the microwave, washing your hands, or brushing your teeth, you can spare 30 seconds of your time to practice this simple balance exercise. The biggest excuse I hear is, "Oh my balance is horrible". Well the secret to better balance is repeated practice, creating lasting muscle memory to keep you steady when it matters.

Is the Problem Really Your Disc?

Are you convinced that your back pain is caused by a disc problem? Here's something to think about: how many people do you know with herniated or bulging discs? Believe it or not, many people don't experience any pain related to the disc. Studies show that over 30% of people over the age of 30 have disc degeneration or bulges visible on MRIs, yet they report no symptoms. If you don't have pain every single day, could it be that your disc isn't the primary source of your discomfort? If you have pain some days and relief on others, it's likely that the issue is mechanical, not structural.

Why Does Resting Make Your Back Worse?

Are you trying to "rest" your way out of back pain? Many of my clients tell me they tried resting, but it only made their pain last longer. Could it be that the *way* you rest—sitting on the couch, lying in bed, with a tablet, using your phone, watching TV—is actually compounding the problem? Studies show that inactivity can weaken your muscles and prolong recovery. What if, instead of resting, you started moving?

Movement is medicine for the spine, and gentle activity helps keep the muscles around the spine engaged and the discs hydrated.

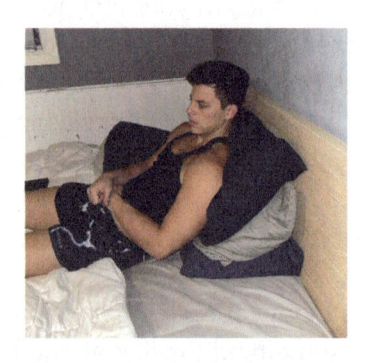

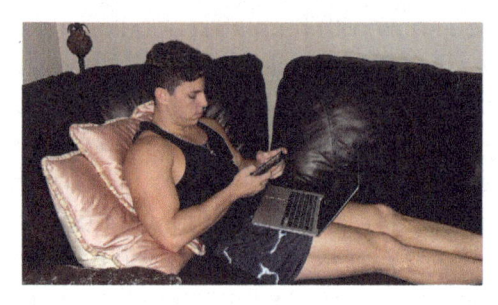

How Often Do You Stand Up and Sit Down?

Has your leg or foot ever gone numb or tingly from sitting too long? Do you know that one of the best exercises for your back is simply standing up and sitting down? At the bare minimum you should be changing postures every 30 minutes. By that, all I mean is stand up and sit back down. It offloads the spine and when you return to sitting the pressure will be on a different muscle or nerve.

I had a client with severe back pain who asked for just one exercise. I recommended standing up and sitting down 10 times with a resistance band around his knees. Not only did he lose 10 pounds in a month, but his back pain improved significantly. One daily victory compounded and led to better decisions. Could adding this simple movement to your daily routine help you manage your pain?

The Secrets About Sciatica

"Sciatica" is probably one of the most overused diagnoses in the physical therapy world. We see it all the time; lower back pain, radiating to the glutes, hip, and down the leg. 9 times out of 10, "sciatica" is not the issue.

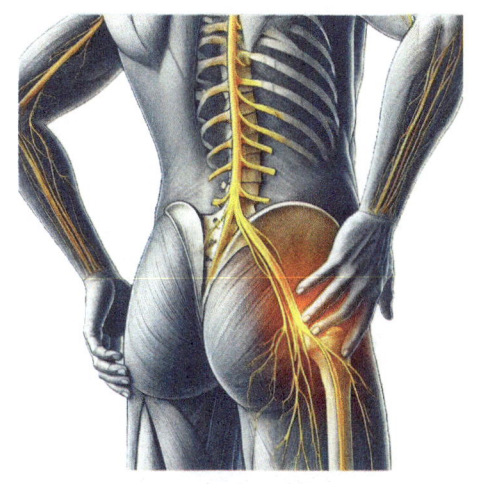

The sciatic nerve is the longest nerve in the body. "Sciatica" is not a condition itself, but rather a symptom of an underlying issue that irritates or compresses the sciatic nerve. The pain is usually described as radiating down the leg, numbness or tingling, weakness, and worse with sitting or standing.

As you've read so far, there are a bunch of other things we do throughout the day that also cause these symptoms. Imagine if you could change 1-2 things on a daily basis to get rid of your sciatica forever?

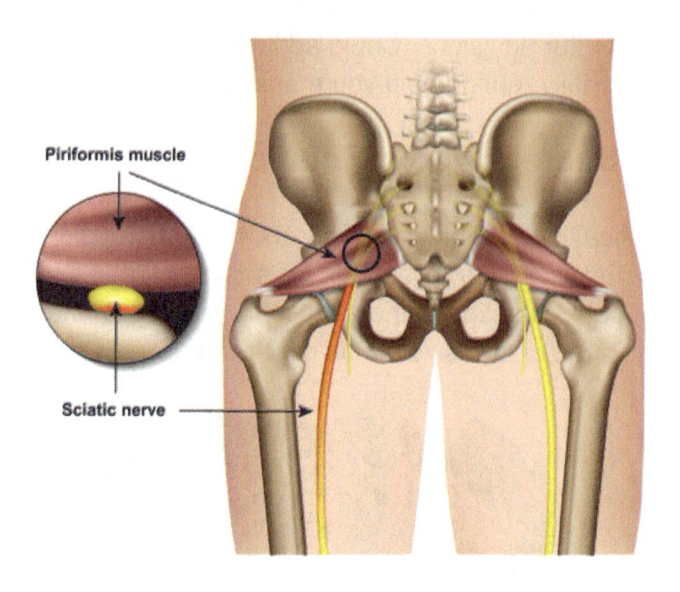

The piriformis muscle, for example, is closely associated with "sciatica" symptoms. The sciatic nerve typically runs beneath, but may pass through the muscle in some individuals. When the piriformis becomes tight, inflamed, or is working insufficiently, it can compress the sciatic nerve. This can cause pain, tingling, or numbness along the sciatic nerve's pathway. Most people would go to the doctor and obtain an MRI to figure out the problem.

Due to our daily habits, many will find disc herniations, spinal stenosis, spondylolisthesis, or degenerative disc disease on imaging, however these changes didn't happen overnight. It's our daily habits that compound, like mileage on a car, and eventually catch up to us.

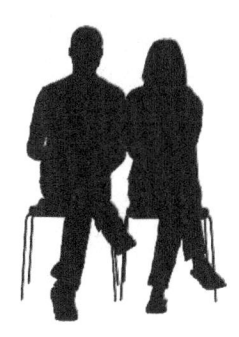

What habits you may ask? Start by uncrossing your legs. When you cross your legs while sitting or laying down, you are causing postural imbalances and strain on the hips, pelvis, and spine. Crossing your legs tilts the pelvis and unevenly distributes your weight, leading to muscle tightness and weakness over time. This position can also restrict blood flow and place unnecessary pressure on the sciatic nerve, potentially exacerbating your pain and causing those nagging referred symptoms down the leg.

Have you ever felt like one leg is longer or shorter than the other? Rarely is this the case from a structural standpoint. Most of the time it is mechanical and happens from repeated movements that cause compensatory pelvic rotation. Crossing your legs has become a default sitting position for many due to postural adaptations, which makes it feel more natural over time. This is not ideal for alignment, rethink how you sit.

We use our muscles every second of every day. It's how we use or abuse them that determines how we feel. You'd be surprised how much pain muscles can cause. What we believe to be nerve pain, can actually be referred pain from irritated or strained muscles. Referred pain is felt in a location other than where the actual problem or injury is occurring.

Here are some diagrams that depict referred pain from muscles that clients often confuse with "sciatica":

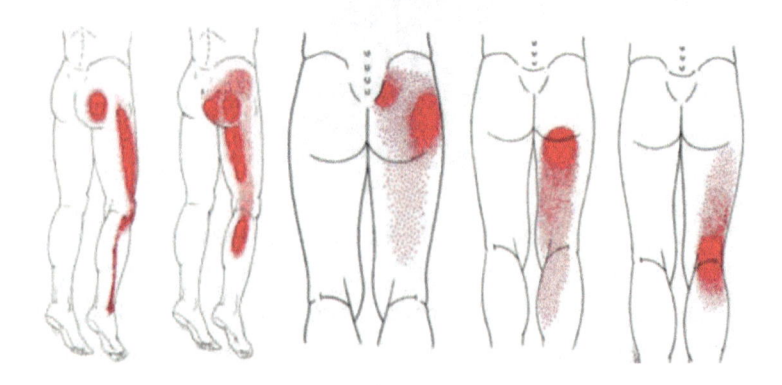

As you can see, the glutes (butt) and hamstring (back of the leg) muscles are a major culprit for mimicking "sciatica" symptoms. Muscles develop trigger points that can cause referred pain that may seem nerve related.

As clinicians, we've had a lot of success treating "sciatica" with dry needling. Dry needling uses an acupuncture-type needle and is used to decrease trigger points. A trigger point is a palpable taut band that reproduces localized or referred pain. Trigger points, known as "knots", may cause restricted range of motion and weakness of a muscle. During treatment, the needle is inserted into a "knot", causing the muscle to twitch, which decreases the muscle tone and often resolves this referred pain. If you've ever considered a cortisone injection for your pain, you should give dry needling a try first!

Is Weak Glute Strength Contributing to Your Pain?

Are your glutes working hard enough to support your spine? Weak glutes are often a hidden cause of back pain, especially as we age. Just because you have big glutes, doesn't mean they're strong. Did you know you have 3 different glutes? Most know about the gluteus maximus, but there is also a gluteus medius and gluteus minimus. All parts of the glute help with hip extension, rotation, and stabilization to help with weight-bearing activities and maintaining an upright posture.

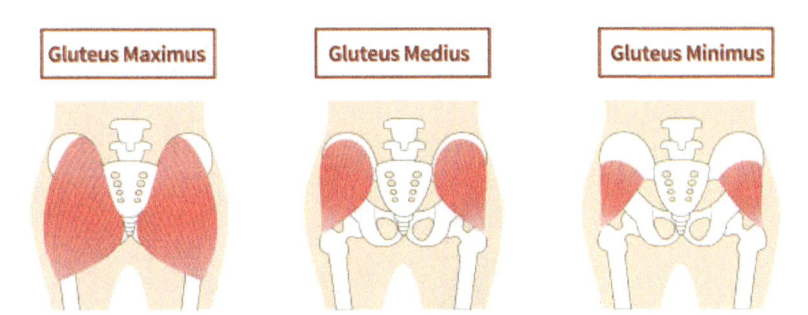

| Gluteus Maximus | Gluteus Medius | Gluteus Minimus |

Most of us spend our day walking in straight lines, firing our quads and hamstrings but neglecting our glutes. If your spine was a baby tree how many wooden posts would hold it up? 3 or 4. When walking in a straight line we're typically activating 2, our quads and our hamstrings. If the baby tree only has 2 posts, when the wind blows the tree would sway and the roots (our muscles) would tighten to try to stabilize leading to imbalances. Could strengthening your glutes help stabilize your back? I've seen countless clients improve their back pain by incorporating glute activation exercises into their routine.

Glutes on the Go: Our Top 3 Favorites

Standing Diagonal Kickbacks

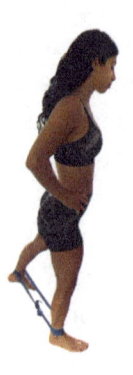

Sit to Stand (with band around knees)

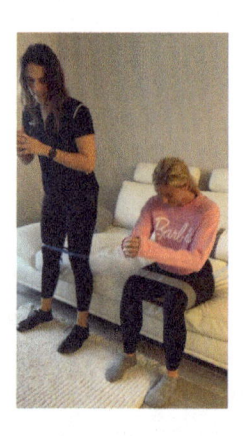

Glute Bridges (with band)

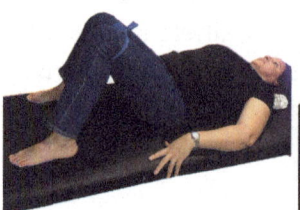

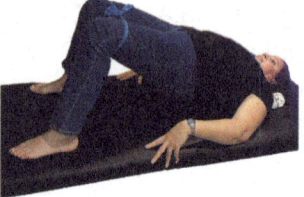

Why Couches Are Killer

Do You Sit in One Spot for Hours?

Could the way you sit on your couch or chair be hurting your spine? Most people sit in the same spot for hours while watching TV or working from home. What if that was the very thing causing your pain? Moving just a little, whether shifting your weight, standing up, or taking a few steps, can be the simple fix your spine needs to feel better.

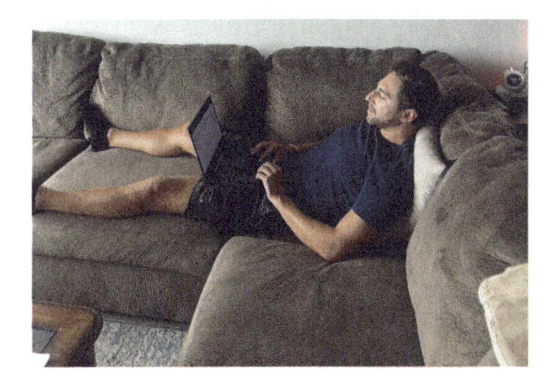

Is There a Good Way to Sit on the Couch?

Do you think there's a good way to sit on a couch? The truth is, couches are killers when it comes to posture. There's really no good way to sit on them without eventually feeling discomfort or pain. Have you ever noticed that the more time you spend on the couch, the worse your back or neck feels? For me, if I spend more than 10 minutes on my couch, I start feeling neck pain, and in 1 to 3 days, it turns into full-blown discomfort or headaches.

One day, I played one hour of Call of Duty and sat at the edge of my bed. I ended up giving myself "sciatica" for 2 days after this one decision.

The only "safe" way I've found to lay on a couch is on your side as if you were side sleeping with a pillow under your neck, between the legs, and between the arms with possibly some support behind the back. Shocker! This is another variation of The Four Pillow Method.

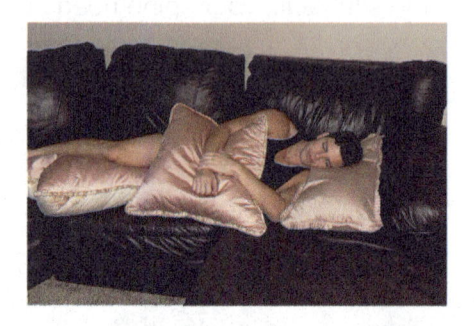

Do You Sit With Your Legs Up?

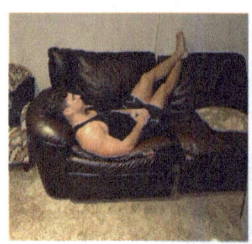

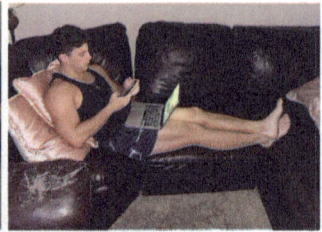

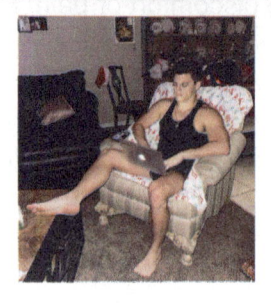

Do you lounge on the L shaped part of your couch? The next time you sit on your couch with your legs up, I want you to pay attention to where the weight goes. Do you feel it settling into your lower back and the hinge joint of your neck? That joint is called the C7 vertebra—it's the one that sticks out at the base of your neck. Over time, this position causes strain and can lead to what we call "dural stretching," which can even increase symptoms like tingling or numbness in your arms or legs. So, if you're wondering why your neck feels stiff after lounging, this could be the reason. Do you ever sit with one leg on a coffee table or something and the other on the floor? This can be a big contributor to low back pain, offsetting the SI joint and lower back mechanics.

The Power of Position Changes: Why Movement Matters

How often do you adjust your position while sitting on the couch? If the answer is "rarely," it's time to rethink your habits.

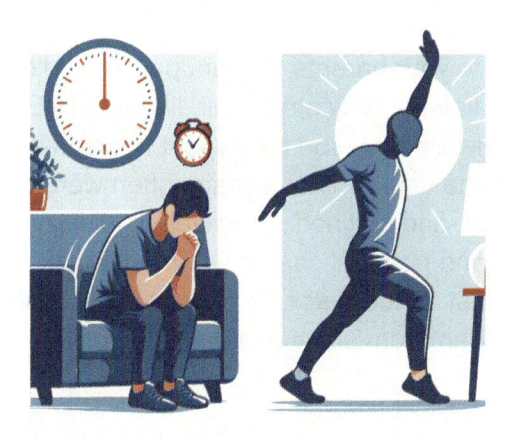

Prolonged sitting in the same posture puts continuous strain on your spine and supporting muscles, leading to stiffness and discomfort. One of the simplest, yet most effective habits you can adopt is setting a timer halfway through a movie or TV show to remind yourself to get up and move. A quick two-minute walk or stretch can help reset your spine, improve circulation, and prevent your body from adapting to poor posture. By incorporating regular position changes, you not only reduce the risk of back pain, but also give your body the variety it craves for healthier, more dynamic movements.

Why We Need to Bring Back Rocking Chairs

Why Were Rocking Chairs So Common?

Have you ever wondered why our grandparents loved rocking chairs? These chairs weren't just for relaxing. They provided constant movement and feedback to the body. Sitting still for too long creates pressure in one spot, which leads to pain. Rocking chairs prevent that by keeping our bodies in motion.

Think back to your parents or grandparents—did your dad or grandpa have a dedicated chair, like a Lazy Boy recliner? There's a reason they spent hours in those chairs rather than the couch. Those chairs often were on a swivel base, rocked, and reclined, or swiveled, allowing for subtle movement and postural changes. Movement is medicine, and that constant feedback from the rocking chair prevented them from staying in one stiff position for too long.

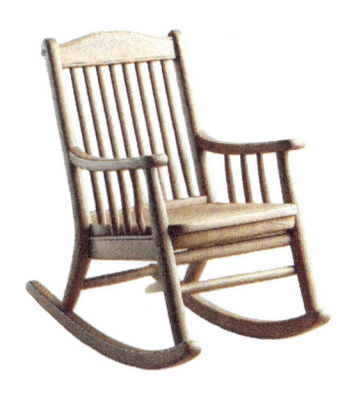

When we think back to our grandparents, everyone had a good old wooden rocking chair. This was for a reason. An object in motion stays in motion. When sitting on a rocking chair you're constantly moving and giving your body gentle feedback and almost providing self joint mobilizations through smooth fluid motions, which can lubricate the joints. Throw away your couch and get a rocking chair today. I typically get my clients to buy a cheap camping rocking chair that they can fold up and put away. Easy, portable, and you can take them camping or to sporting events.

Could Rocking Chairs Help Solve Modern Pain Problems?

In my experience, the more I work with people, the more I realize that a good old-fashioned rocking chair could solve many modern pain problems. It keeps the body gently moving, distributing weight evenly and avoiding prolonged pressure on any one part of the spine. Could a rocking chair be a better solution for long periods of sitting compared to your couch or desk chair?

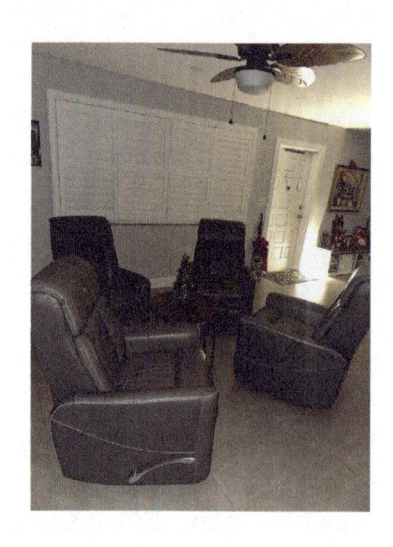

What About Those Fancy Desk Chairs and Cushions?

Have you invested in expensive desk chairs or seat cushions, hoping they'd solve your back pain? While some of these options are helpful, they often don't fix the root cause: staying still for too long. I once had a client who bought all kinds of ergonomic cushions for his new car, thinking it would help with his back pain, but he still had pain every time he drove. When I watched how he sat, I realized the problem wasn't the chair—it was how he was sitting. His elbow was propped up on his lap, shifting his spine, which was the real issue. As you now know, leaning is a huge problem, especially when sitting.

Desk Life

The same movement principles apply to those who work at a desk or spend long periods sitting. If you don't have a standing desk, I highly recommend investing in one. They're relatively affordable these days, often around $120. But you don't have to stand all day to make a difference. The key is movement! Adjust the height of your desk by a few degrees every 20 minutes. If a standing desk isn't an option, move your chair height and position more often. Your body continuously craves movement, even the smallest changes will save your spine.

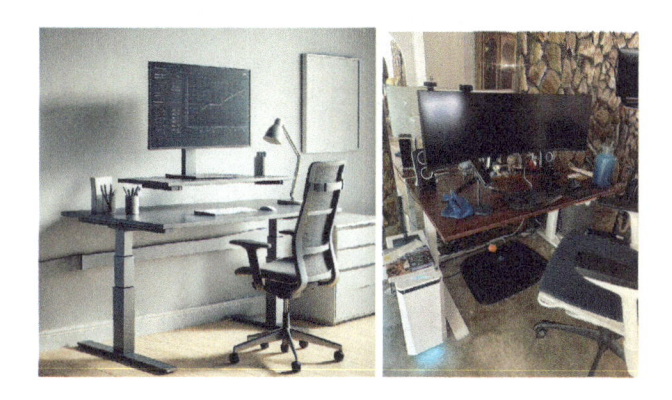

How Ergonomic Tools Can Help

If you're going to stand, use an ergonomic mat. Studies show they can reduce fatigue by up to 50%.[10] Some ergonomic mats even come with built-in balls or ridges so you can roll out your feet or stretch while standing. These mats improve proprioceptive awareness and encourage constant micro-movements, helping you avoid stiffness and pain. I'll admit, when I was writing this book, I developed a little sacral pain because my feet weren't in contact with the floor. Lesson learned!

Under desk bicycles or treadmills are also great to have. I envision a future where desks have resistance bands or cables attached to them for exercise while you work.

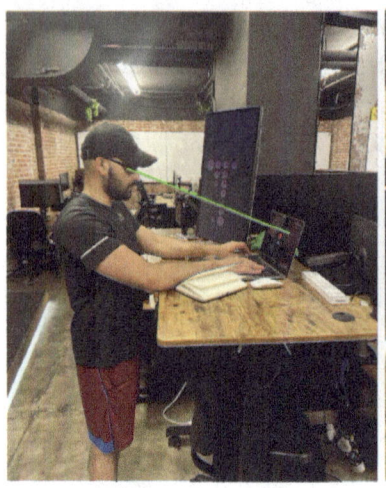

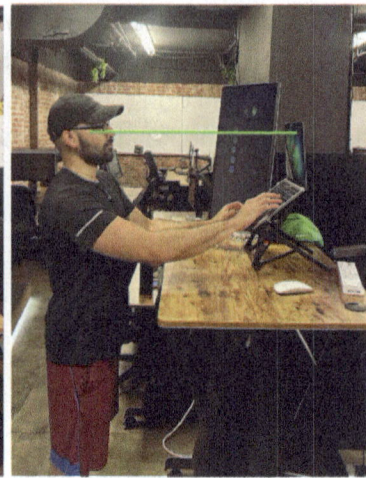

Remember, even if you have a standing desk you still need a laptop stand.

Is Biking Making Your Back Pain Worse?

I had a client who reported back pain that started following an increase in working out. She was very disappointed since she was trying to move more and hadn't had back pain this bad before. I asked her what type of exercise she was doing and she mentioned biking. I asked if she did any warm up or had any biker shorts. After just one Slight Motion session and introducing proper biker shorts, she reported a significant decrease in pain.

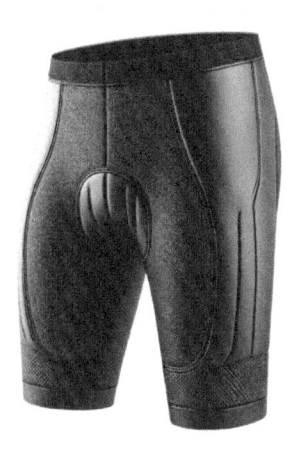

Are you someone who has started biking to lose weight or improve your fitness? Biking is an excellent form of cardio, but not without its risks—especially for your back. Many people report back pain after biking, and most of the time, it's because they aren't wearing the right gear. If you're biking for more than 10 minutes without wearing biker shorts, you're likely putting unnecessary strain on your back. Biker shorts provide the padding and support needed to avoid discomfort during long rides. So, if you're experiencing back pain from biking, consider investing in the right gear.

Key Takeaways on Movement

Movement isn't just good for your back—it's essential for your whole body. Whether you're sitting at a desk, driving, or relaxing at home, making small adjustments to your posture throughout the day can prevent pain from building up. From using a standing desk to wearing biker shorts while cycling, these minor changes can make a major difference in how your body feels.

Remember: A little movement goes a long way.

What if We Made Movement Part of Everyday Life?

Have you ever thought about how efficient it would be if movement were part of everything we do? What if desks came with resistance bands, cables, and columns attached to them, allowing you to move while you work? Imagine airports where people are doing banded workouts in line, making the most of their time while waiting for flights. Movement isn't just medicine for your back—it's medicine for your whole body.

How Can You Incorporate More Movement at Home?

Do you have small opportunities to add movement to your day at home? Think about the time you spend on the couch, at your desk, or in front of the TV. Could you add some gentle movements, rocking, or even just walking around during commercial breaks? These small, frequent actions can go a long way in preventing stiffness and pain from building up.

Back Squats, Core Work, and Protecting Your Spine

Should You Be Doing Back Squats?

Do you regularly do back squats in your workout routine? If so, you might want to reconsider. The main goal of keeping our spine healthy is decompressing the discs, not compressing them with heavy loads. Think about it, why would you want to put 275 pounds of weight through your spine, essentially stacking all that pressure on top of your head?

If you have a disc bulge or a herniation, you're already dealing with disc compression. Back squats only add more pressure, which can aggravate existing spinal issues.

The load on the spine during a back squat can be substantial. Studies estimate that the lumbar spine experiences compressive forces of 6 to 10 times body weight depending on the weight lifted, squat depth, and form.[11] For example, if someone weighs 200 lbs and squats with 300 lbs, the spine could endure 3,000–5,000 lbs of force. Proper technique, core stability, and load management are essential to minimize injury risks and evenly distribute force across muscles and joints.

What Are Better Alternatives to Back Squats?

Front squats could be a better alternative if you still want to incorporate squats into your routine. Front squats shift the weight forward, placing less direct load on your spine and allowing for a more upright position, which decreases the risk of spinal compression. But even better than squats might be focusing on core stabilization exercises that protect your spine rather than loading it with excessive weight.

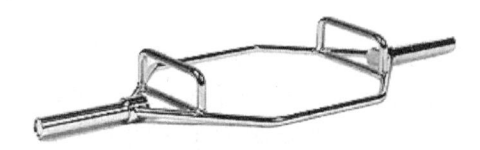

Does your gym have a Hex Bar? Squatting with a Hex Bar allows you to load the appropriate weight and maintains your body in a more functional position. Why do we squat? We do it all day. Everytime we sit in a chair or pick up something from the floor, we're squatting.

"But my Doctor says squats are bad for me."

It's one of the most functional, most foundational movements we know. Squats aren't bad for you. Squatting with bad mechanics or too heavy of a load is bad for you and can cause long-term spinal damage.

Are You Still Doing Sit-Ups?

If you're not an athlete or fighter, why are you still doing sit-ups? Sit-ups place unnecessary strain on your spine, compressing the discs as you repeatedly curl your body forward. We already spend most of our day fighting to stand up tall, counteracting the effects of poor posture. Adding sit-ups into the mix only reinforces the very angles we're trying to avoid. Strengthening your core in these compromised positions can lead to long-term back pain and disc issues.

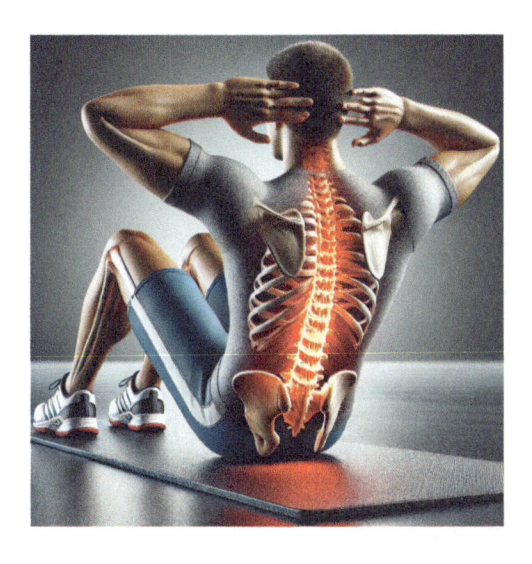

What Are Better Core Exercises?

Instead of sit-ups and Russian twists, consider these core exercises that provide stability without compressing the spine:

Planks: Holding a plank for even just one second a day can make you feel accomplished. Ideally, try to hold it for longer, but start small if needed. Planks are a great way to build core strength while keeping your spine in a neutral position.

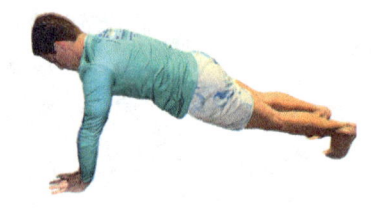

Side Planks: Holding a side plank for 30 seconds on each side before your workout primes your core for lateral stability and stabilizes the muscles around your spine. This helps you maintain proper alignment and control during dynamic movements.

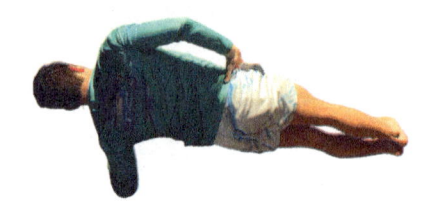

Suitcase Carries: This highly functional exercise mimics real-life movements, like carrying groceries, bags, or even kids. Since we perform these actions daily, it makes sense to train your body to handle them efficiently. To perform a suitcase carry, hold a weight in one hand and walk steadily, focusing on engaging your core and resisting the natural tendency to lean or tilt toward the weighted side. This exercise strengthens your core, improves stability, and helps reduce unnecessary strain on your spine, making everyday tasks easier and safer.

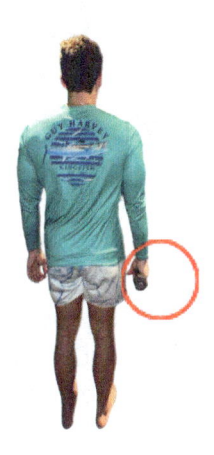

Bird Dog: If you can get on all fours, Bird Dog is one of my favorite core exercises. It trains your body for multiplanar stability, meaning your core has to stay strong in various directions. This exercise strengthens your spine-supporting muscles while improving balance and coordination.

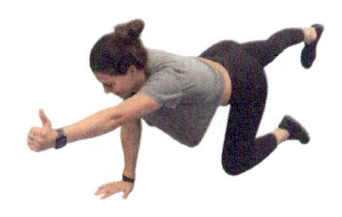

Pallof Presses: A safer alternative to Russian twists, Pallof presses engage the core through anti-rotation. By resisting movement instead of forcing it, you build core strength while protecting your spine from the twisting and torquing that can lead to injury.

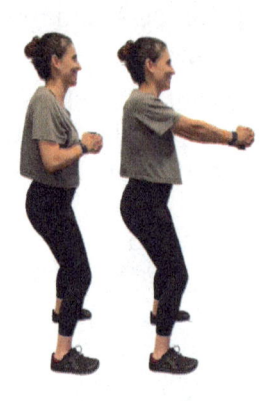

Dead Bug: If getting on your hands and knees for a Bird Dog is difficult, try the Dead Bug exercise. It's a similar stabilizing movement, but it's done while lying on your back, making it more accessible for those with mobility limitations. Like Bird Dog, it focuses on core stability without loading the spine.

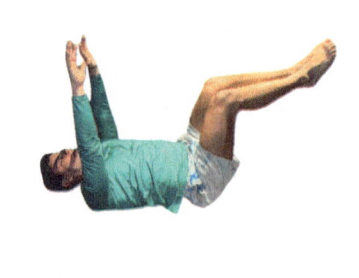

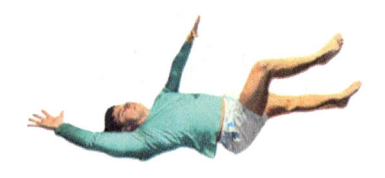

Protecting Your Lumbar Spine For Life

Your lumbar spine is the powerhouse of your body's movements, providing the strength and flexibility needed for everyday activities like bending, lifting, and twisting. But with great power comes great responsibility. Neglecting the health of your lower back can lead to chronic pain and limited mobility. By understanding how small habits, posture, and daily movements affect your lumbar spine, you can take proactive steps to protect it. Whether it's through strengthening exercises, better ergonomics and sitting postures, or simply learning to move with intention, investing in your lumbar health ensures a stronger foundation for everything you do. Remember, small adjustments lead to big improvements, so start building better habits today to support a lifetime of healthy movement.

Chapter 9
Hip Habits

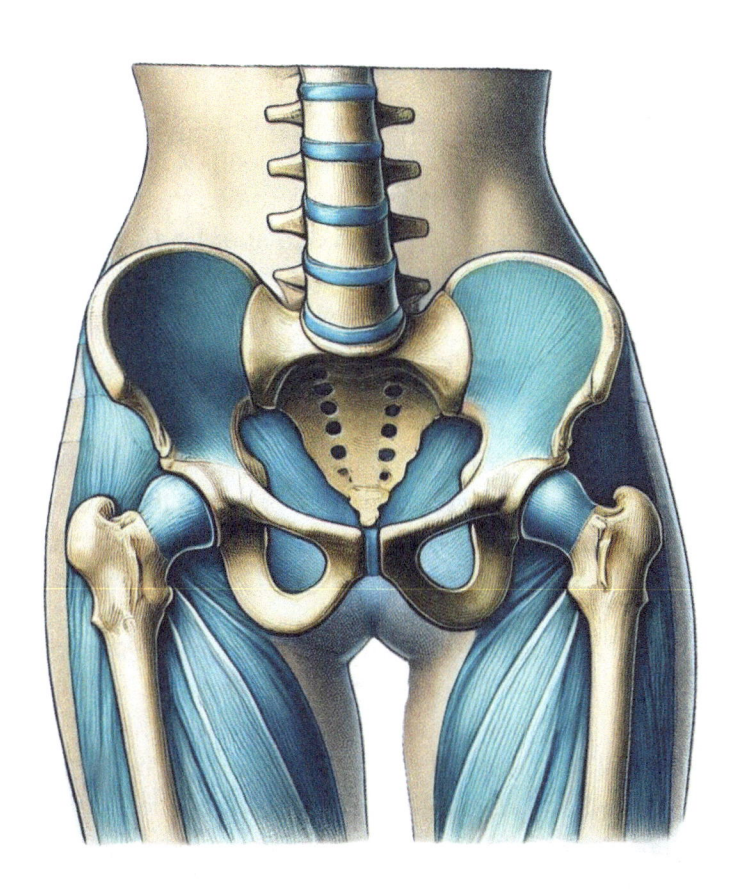

Hip Habits

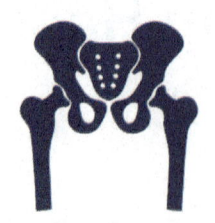

Hip pain is a common issue that affects people of all ages, from the highly active to the more sedentary. Have you ever wondered where your hip pain comes from? Most people assume it's due to aging or a specific injury, but did you know that it often stems from the small, repetitive actions and habits we perform every day? These seemingly insignificant habits can lead to muscle imbalances, joint strain, and persistent pain.

In this chapter, we'll dive into real-life examples of how small adjustments can alleviate hip pain and the importance of becoming more aware of your daily actions to prevent and manage hip discomfort.

Your hips are the unsung heroes of movement, providing stability, power, and mobility for everything from walking and sitting to climbing stairs and athletic performance. As the central link between your upper and lower body, the hips absorb and distribute forces, ensuring smooth and efficient movement. Yet, many of us develop habits—like prolonged sitting, poor posture, or uneven weight distribution—that place unnecessary strain on the hip joints and surrounding muscles. Over time, these habits can lead to tightness, imbalances, and even pain, affecting how we move and feel.

The Million-Dollar MRI Myth

"Your MRI shows significant wear and tear.

At your age, this is to be expected..."

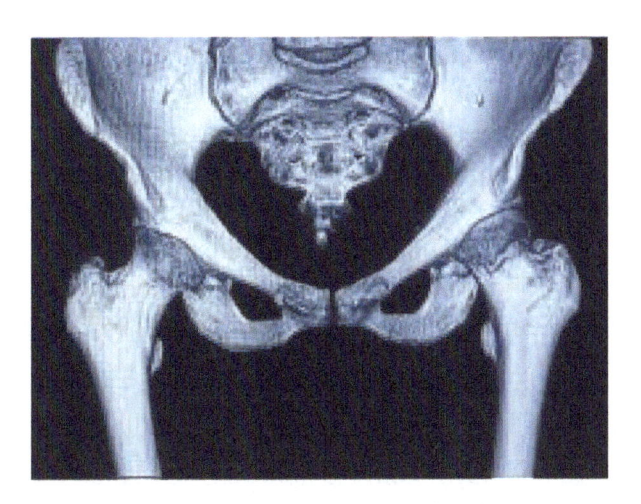

If you've heard these words from your doctor, you're not alone.

Here's the shocking truth: in a groundbreaking study of people with NO hip pain, researchers found[12]:

- 69% had labral tears
- 24% had cartilage damage
- 20% had bone spurs
- And numerous other "abnormalities"

That's right. These people were living completely pain-free lives despite having the same "problems" that might have led your doctor to recommend you surgery.

These findings reveal that structural abnormalities can exist without causing pain, suggesting that not every visible issue on an MRI or scan is necessarily problematic. In fact, anatomical variations are often more common than you might think. Everyone's body is uniquely structured. Factors like natural variations in pelvic tilt, the shape and depth of the hip joint, and overall alignment can influence MRI results without necessarily causing symptoms. Anatomical differences are common and part of what makes each body unique. These natural variations, such as differences in pelvic tilt or hip joint shape, do not always cause symptoms or indicate a problem. Rather than viewing all 'abnormalities' as harmful, it's important to recognize them as part of the natural diversity of human anatomy.

For instance, one review found that 37% of over 2,000 young hips had asymptomatic deformities, with 54.8% of those cases in athletes compared to 23.1% in non-athletes. In a study of collegiate football players, 95% of the 134 hips analyzed had at least one sign of hip impingement, and 77% had more than one sign. Even more broadly, hip impingement is estimated to affect around 30% of the general population and up to 75% of athletes.[13-15]

These statistics underscore a crucial point. Many people, especially athletes, live pain-free despite common structural "abnormalities" like hip impingement. The presence of these variations on an MRI doesn't necessarily indicate a need for intervention or surgery.

How Do You Sit?

Have you ever considered how your sitting posture affects your hip health? The way you sit plays a significant role in hip pain, particularly when it comes to leg positioning.

Understanding "Manspreading"

The term "manspreading" refers to the way some men sit with their legs spread wide apart, particularly in public space. While it may be seen as a social phenomenon, this sitting posture has a physiological basis rooted in hip anatomy and function. Men naturally tend to sit with their legs apart because it aligns with the structure of the male pelvis and the position of the hip joints. The male pelvis is generally narrower than the female pelvis, and sitting with the legs slightly apart can help reduce tension in the hip joints and the surrounding muscles.

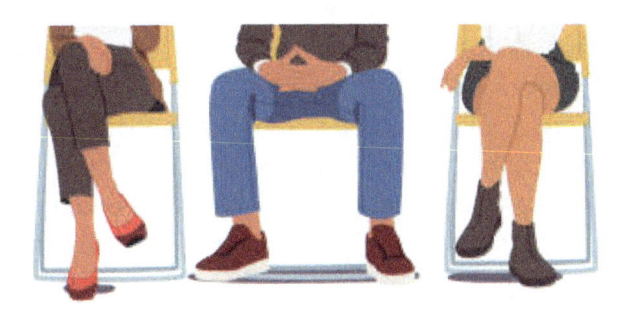

The Problem with Crossing Legs

On the other hand, crossing the legs or sitting with them closer together, particularly with the legs tightly crossed at the knees, can create significant strain on the hips. Unevenly bearing your weight through your pelvis and hips can lead to hip and even lower back pain. This position forces the hip joint into an internally rotated position, which can lead to hip impingement—a condition where the bones of the hip joint rub against each other or pinch the surrounding soft tissues. Over time, this impingement can cause pain, stiffness, and even contribute to more serious issues like labral tears or arthritis.

How Do You Stand?

A client came to us with persistent hip pain. He was doing everything right, or so he thought. He had a body pillow in front of him and behind him when sleeping. As discussed in the pillow talk section body pillows can be problematic. The body pillow behind him might've been too big to tuck in. He would hook his right leg up while keeping his left leg straight which might've been a contributor as well. He worked at the wrong desk height, without a standing desk, although he did have an ergonomic mat with a foot roller on it. We fixed all these things and the pain improved.

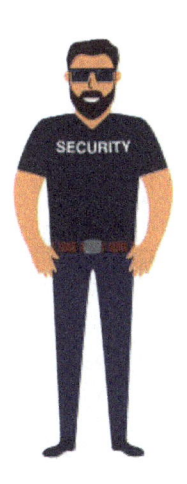

Through the Slight Motion Method and awareness of all the little things we created he realized when standing at a bar or stationary he would stand to one side putting most of his weight on his right hip without fully offloading the left leg. We see this often as a contributor and educate our clients to stand in the "Bodyguard Position", with weight equally distributed between both legs. If you've noticed, bodyguards stand with a specific posture because they typically have to stay in that position for an extended period of time.

If this seems unrealistic for you, you can modify it into a balance exercise by fully shifting your weight onto the leg you're favoring, practicing single-leg balance. To make it more dynamic, try a staggered stance and gently shift your weight from your front to back leg. This subtle movement engages your hips and glutes, helping stabilize your pelvis and preventing impingement or misalignment on one side. There are always simple ways to improve the movements we perform every day.

Hip Impingement and Pain

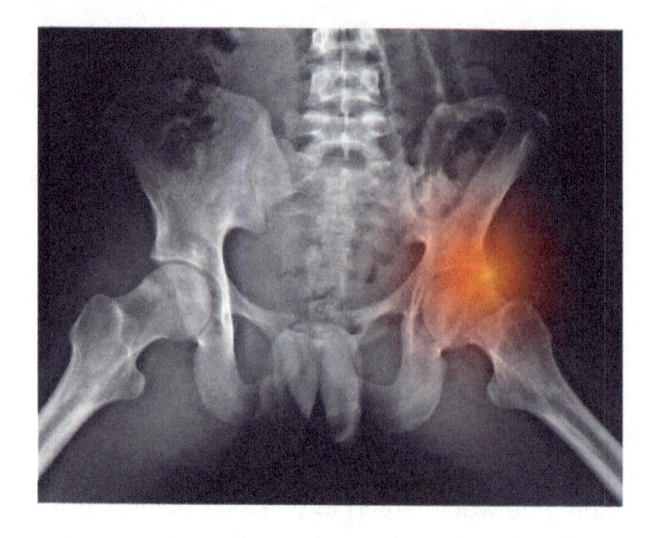

Hip impingement, also known as femoroacetabular impingement (FAI), occurs when there is abnormal contact between the femoral head and the acetabulum (the socket of the hip). This abnormal contact can be exacerbated by sitting positions that force the hips into unnatural angles, such as crossing the legs tightly or sleeping without a pillow between the knees, as discussed in the Pillow Talk chapter. When the hip is internally rotated for extended periods, it puts stress on the labrum (the cartilage that lines the hip socket) and the surrounding muscles, leading to pain and discomfort.

It is often found that people who sit with their legs crossed or in positions that promote internal hip rotation are at a higher risk of developing hip impingement. This condition is particularly prevalent among people who spend long hours sitting at desks, in cars, or in other sedentary positions.

The Benefits of a Neutral Sitting Position

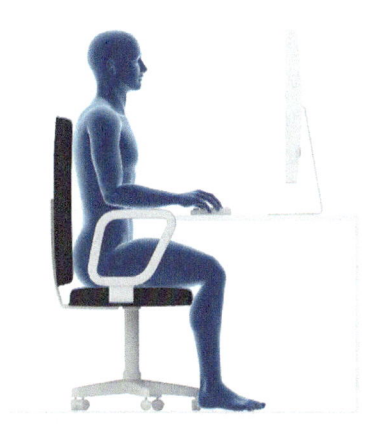

To prevent hip impingement and reduce pain, most recommend adopting a neutral sitting position. This means sitting with your feet flat on the floor, knees at a 90-degree angle, and hips aligned with the rest of your body. Keeping your legs uncrossed and slightly apart helps maintain proper hip alignment and reduces the strain on the joints and surrounding muscles. I'm sure you've heard this all before but I think this is where a lot of people go wrong. There's no perfect posture, your best posture is your next posture. Any position for too long is dangerous, the key is constant movement. We've discovered that movement is medicine and we want to constantly be adjusting chair height. Set a reminder to adjust your chair height or stand up for a quick stretch every 20-30 minutes.

For men, sitting with the legs slightly apart (within a comfortable and socially acceptable range) can help maintain this neutral position, reducing the risk of hip impingement. For both men and women, being mindful of leg positioning and avoiding prolonged periods of crossing the legs can prevent unnecessary stress on the hips. We know it is unrealistic to say to NEVER cross your legs when sitting, but we hope that by bringing this habit to light, it will allow you to sit like this for maybe two minutes instead of two hours.

Why Your Best Posture Is Your Next Posture

Rachel, an online yoga instructor, came to me confused and frustrated. Despite her excellent flexibility and posture awareness, she was experiencing persistent hip pain. "I don't understand," she said during our first meeting. "I maintain perfect posture all day. I never cross my legs, I sit up straight, I do everything right." Ironically, that was the problem.

Like many of my clients, Rachel had fallen into what I call the "perfect posture trap". The belief that if we just find the right position and maintain it, our pain will disappear. She'd even bought an expensive ergonomic chair and set timers to check her alignment throughout the day.

"Show me how you sit during your workday," I requested.

She demonstrated her "perfect" position: feet flat on the floor, knees at exactly 90 degrees, back straight as an arrow. She held this position religiously, afraid that any deviation would cause pain.

"And how long do you maintain this position?"

"As long as I can," she replied proudly. "Sometimes for hours."

Here's what research and clinical experience have taught me:

- There is no "perfect" posture
- Your best posture is your next posture
- Movement variety is more important than any perfect position
- Even the "ideal" position becomes problematic when held too long

I shared a simple experiment with Rachel. "For the next week, instead of maintaining one 'perfect' position, I want you to change your chair height slightly every hour. Sit in a variety of positions throughout the day. Stand up occasionally. Just keep moving."

She looked skeptical. "But won't that make my alignment worse?"

One week later, Rachel called me, excitement in her voice. "My hip pain... it's almost gone. I never realized how much tension I was creating by trying to maintain perfect posture."

This doesn't mean we should ignore posture completely. But rather than thinking of posture as a fixed position to maintain, think of it as a dynamic range of movements to explore.

Set a timer for every 30 minutes and try this:

- Adjust your chair height slightly
- Change your leg position
- Stand up and move for 1-2 minutes

One month after our initial session, Rachel had transformed her approach to sitting. "I used to think movement was something you did during exercise," she told me. "Now I realize it's something we should do all day long."

The biggest lesson from Rachel's case wasn't about finding the right position - it was about learning to let go of the idea that any single position could be "right" for very long. Our bodies crave movement variety.

Unconscious Habits: The Culprits of Pain

Many people unknowingly sit in positions that can contribute to hip pain. Sitting with one leg tucked under you or propping a foot up on the chair can also create imbalances in the muscles and joints.

A client of mine experienced severe hip pain that wouldn't go away despite trying various treatments. When I visited her home, I discovered that she did most of her work sitting on bar stools with no laptop stand, causing her legs to dangle. This position put a strain on her hips and lower back, exacerbating her pain. After advising her to switch to a more supportive chair and ensure her feet were flat on the floor, her hip pain began to subside.

The Occupational Health and Safety Administration (OSHA) reports that prolonged sitting in poor ergonomic positions is a well-documented risk factor for developing musculoskeletal disorders, including hip pain.[16] Ensuring that your feet are in contact with the floor while sitting helps provide necessary feedback and support, reducing the risk of pain.

When Work Hurts: A Case of Desk-Related Hip Pain

"I can barely walk," Maria winced as she tried to stand from her office chair. At 34 years old, she was leading a major software project, but something as simple as getting up had become an ordeal. "The pain... it's like a knife in my hip.

Three doctors have suggested surgery for a possible labral tear."

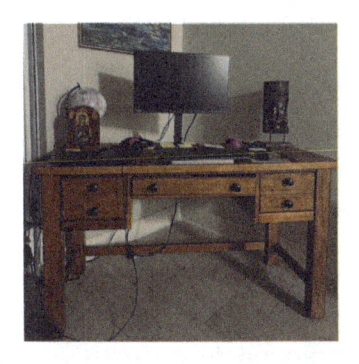

As she settled back into her chair at her antique desk, I noticed something interesting. There was a beautiful wooden beam running across the bottom, about eight inches off the ground. Without thinking, she lifted her feet to rest on it.

"How long do you work like this?" I asked.

"Usually four or five hours, but with this project deadline..." She looked down. "Probably nine or ten hours some days. But it's comfortable! The beam is at just the right height."

That word - "comfortable" - often raises red flags in my practice. What feels comfortable in the moment can create lasting problems over time.

"Try something for me," I suggested. "Sit how you normally would, feet on the beam." She did. "Now, notice your lower back. Are you leaning forward slightly?"

She started to say no, then stopped. "Oh... I guess I am. Just a little though."

"That 'little' lean, multiplied by ten hours, multiplied by weeks of project work..."

Her eyes widened with recognition.

I called a respected colleague for a second opinion. He examined her and confirmed what he believed to be a labral tear. "The MRI shows some irregularities," he explained. "Surgery might be your best option."

But something didn't add up. The timing of her pain's onset matched perfectly with her project's increased workload. Her symptoms worsened during workdays and improved on weekends.

We made two simple changes right there in her office:

1. Removed the temptation to rest her feet on the beam
2. Set a timer to stand up every 20 minutes

"That's it?" she asked skeptically.

"Try it for two weeks," I suggested. "If it doesn't help, we can always pursue other options."

Three weeks later, I saw her walking confidently between meetings in heels. "No surgery!" she called out. "Who knew a desk beam could cause so much trouble?"

Sometimes the most significant pain has the simplest cause. While imaging might show irregularities, as it did in Maria's case, these findings don't always tell the whole story. Her experience taught me something crucial: in our modern world, we need to look at how people live, not just at their medical images.

When Zoom Calls Created a Pain Crisis

Mark, a 55-year-old lawyer, was struggling with persistent left hip pain. He was considering a hip replacement, but trying to hold off. When we sat down in his office, he was visibly frustrated. Despite his efforts to stay healthy and comfortable while working, a pain in his hip had worsened over time, seemingly without reason. Our conversation soon revealed that this wasn't just a case of long hours at a desk but something much more subtle.

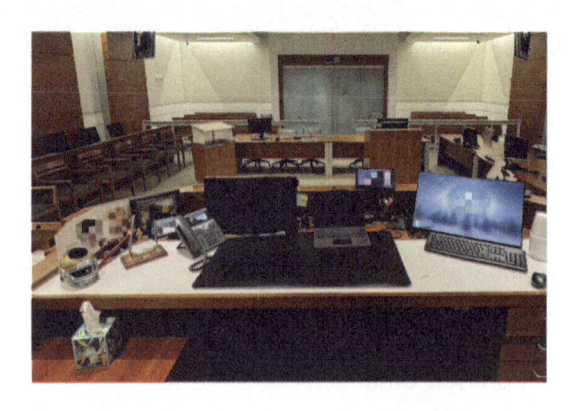

As we talked, something caught my eye. Each time his computer chimed with a notification, he reflexively twisted to his right, his left knee angling inward as he turned to his second monitor—the one dedicated to his endless Zoom calls.

"How many virtual meetings do you have in a typical day?" I asked, noticing the subtle shift he made each time he repositioned himself in his chair.

"Oh, probably 2-3," he replied, turning right again as yet another notification sounded. "Sometimes they're back-to-back, lasting hours."

It wasn't long before I saw the real culprit. Mark's beautiful desk, with its traditional, ornate cubby underneath, was a classic lawyer's setup—but it left his legs no room to move freely. Each time he turned for a Zoom call, his left knee had nowhere to go except inward. His left knee folded inward, while his torso rotated to the right. This seemingly minor twist was putting constant stress on his hip, a strain repeated hundreds of times a week.

"Mark," I said, "show me how you position yourself when you start a Zoom call."

He turned, and there it was—the habitual twist. His left knee collapsed inward, trapped by the desk's design, while his torso rotated to the right. It was a small movement, but when repeated so frequently, it became a source of deep-seated pain.

"But this is just how I set up for calls," he protested. "And it's only turning to look at a screen."

Understanding Repetitive Strain

What Mark didn't realize was that even minor movements, when repeated enough, can become significant sources of pain:

- 2-3 meetings a day
- Each lasting 30-60 minutes
- Frequent rotation to the right
- Left knee forced inward
- Hip kept in a subtle but constant misalignment

The Simple Fix

We made two small adjustments that day:

1. **Repositioned his monitor** directly in front of him, eliminating the need to twist.
2. **Removed the cubby panel** under his desk, freeing his legs and allowing his body to move naturally.

Three weeks later, Mark called me, almost amazed. "I can't believe it was that simple," he said. "My hip pain is nearly gone. I didn't realize how much I was twisting until I stopped doing it."

Try This: A Workspace Audit

Mark's story underscores the importance of examining our daily routines. If you're experiencing discomfort, take a moment to do a "meeting audit" of your workspace:

- **Where is your screen during video calls?** Is it centered, or are you constantly turning?
    - Screen Position: During video calls, is your screen centered, or are you constantly turning?
- **Are your legs restricted?** Check if anything under your desk limits movement.
    - Leg freedom: check for any barriers under your desk that restrict natural movement
- **How often do you repeat the same posture?** Small movements add up over time.
    - Repetitive Postures: Identify minor motions you repeat throughout the day; these add up over time!

Mark's case showed me that even the most professional-looking setups can force us into harmful postures. His impressive, traditional desk—designed for looks—was actually a contributor to his pain. This experience is a reminder that adapting our spaces for technology, like positioning a screen for video calls, can have surprising effects on our health. Now, whenever I see clients with hip pain, one of my first questions is about their video call setup. As Mark told me during a follow-up, "I thought I needed physical therapy or surgery. Turns out, I just needed to turn my monitor."

The Barstool Mystery: Height, Habits, and Hidden Pain

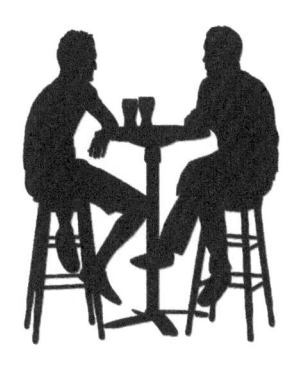

Claire, a 38-year-old freelance writer, came to me after months of unexplained hip pain. She'd tried everything - physical therapy, massage, stretching routines - but nothing seemed to help. "Some days I can barely walk," she told me during our first phone call. "And no one can tell me why."

When I arrived at her home office, the mystery began to unravel. Claire had created what she thought was the perfect workspace: a beautiful high-top table with trendy bar stools, overlooking her garden. "I love working here," she explained, perching on one of the stools. "The view is amazing, and it feels so modern."

But as she sat there, I noticed something crucial - her feet dangling several inches above the floor, unconsciously swinging as she worked. No amount of scenic views could make up for what this was doing to her body.

"How long do you usually work here?" I asked, watching how she shifted her weight every few minutes without even realizing it.

"Oh, most of the day," she replied. "I try to get up sometimes, but when I'm in the flow of writing..." She gestured to her laptop, which sat directly on the high-top table, forcing her to hunch slightly forward.

When our feet can't reach the floor:

- Our body loses its base of support, which makes it harder for core muscles to stabilize the torso
- Hip flexors remain in constant tension
- Lower back compensates for instability
- Blood flow to legs is restricted
- Proprioceptive feedback is compromised

"Claire," I said, "show me how your hips feel after sitting here for an hour." She slid off the stool, wincing as her feet hit the floor. The movement told me everything I needed to know. Her hip flexors were so tight they were affecting her whole walking pattern.

"But it's such a beautiful setup," she protested when I explained the problem. Like many of my clients, she'd prioritized aesthetics over ergonomics, not realizing the two don't have to be mutually exclusive.

We made two immediate changes:

1. Moved her workspace to a proper-height desk with a supportive chair
2. Added a laptop stand to bring her screen to eye level

"But what about my view?" she asked. "We'll keep the high-top setup for short tasks and breaks," I explained. "But for long working sessions, your body needs proper support."

Claire called me, excitement in her voice. "I can't believe it was the bar stools all along," she said. "I've been blaming stress, age, even my mattress - but it was just my feet not touching the floor!"

Studies show that proper foot support while sitting is crucial for:

- Maintaining pelvic alignment
- Supporting natural spine curves
- Enabling proper muscle activation
- Promoting healthy circulation

A month after making these changes, Claire's hip pain had virtually disappeared. She kept her beloved high-top table, but used it differently - for coffee breaks, standing laptop work with laptop on a stand, and short tasks, not eight-hour workdays.

"The funny thing is," she told me during our follow-up, "I didn't even realize my feet were dangling. It's amazing how we can get used to something that's literally hurting us every day." Sometimes the cause of our pain isn't what we're doing wrong, but what we've gotten used to. Claire's story reminds us that comfort and familiarity don't always equal health.

Take a "height audit" of where you sit:

- Are your feet fully supported when you sit?
  - If not, adjust your seat height or use a footrest
    - Vary the seat height periodically
- Can you place your feet flat on the floor?
- Does your seat height match your work surface?
- How long do you maintain any given position?

Hidden in Plain Sight: How a Toilet Paper Holder Created Constant Pain

It was during a summer visit to my college roommate, Michelle, that I stumbled upon a surprising answer to her persistent hip pain. We hadn't seen each other in months, but I noticed immediately how she winced slightly with certain movements. "Three weeks of physical therapy," she sighed over coffee. "And I'm still not better."

As we spent the afternoon reminiscing, Michelle described her struggle. Multiple physical therapy sessions, dedicated stretching, even a new mattress hadn't brought any real improvement. She was convinced that her pain was just another mystery she'd have to live with. Little did either of us know, the solution was hiding in plain sight.

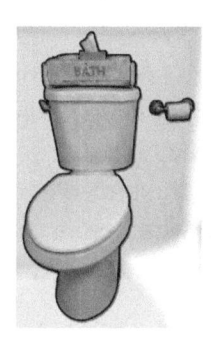

Then came the moment that changed everything. I used her bathroom and suddenly understood what her Physical Therapist had missed. The toilet paper holder was mounted on the wall behind the toilet, requiring an awkward twist to reach it. It seemed insignificant at first glance—something so small that she would never think twice about it. But as I left the bathroom, I had a realization.

"Michelle," I asked when I came out, "how many times a day do you think you reach for that toilet paper?"

She looked confused. "I don't know... maybe six or seven times? Why?"

"And how long have you lived in this apartment?"

"About eight months... around when the hip pain started." Her eyes widened as she made the connection.

Think about it:

- Six or seven twists every day
- 365 days a year
- Each twist forcing the hip into an uncomfortable, impinging position
- The movement repeated without thought

This wasn't what started her pain, but it was like picking a scab. It prevented her hip from fully healing. Each time her body started to recover, this small, unconscious twist irritated her hip again, restarting the cycle of pain. Michelle was skeptical. "It's just reaching for toilet paper," she said. Like many clients, she found it hard to believe that something so minor could have such a lasting impact. But we tried a simple change—placing a freestanding toilet paper holder in front of her instead. Two weeks later, she texted me: "My hip pain is finally starting to stay away. I've gone days without feeling the pain, I can't believe we didn't think of this sooner."

Key Lesson

This experience taught me a valuable lesson about pain: it's not always the big movements that keep us hurting. Often, it's the small, repeated actions that fly under our radar. We don't notice them because they become automatic, but over time, they can have a significant impact.

A Simple Practice: The Movement Audit

Michelle's story is a reminder that sometimes, healing requires us to question even our most basic habits. Take a moment to do a "movement audit" of your daily routine:

- What repetitive movements do you make without thinking?
- Are there awkward reaches or twists in your daily routine? (you do throughout the day)
- What "automatic" movements could you adjust to support your body?

Michelle later shared that she's more aware of these little movements now, noticing patterns in her daily activities she hadn't considered before. "I never thought something as simple as reaching for toilet paper could affect my whole life," she said. "Now I notice these little movements everywhere." Her story reminds us all to look closer at the habits that may be hiding in plain sight.

My Own Battle with Hip Pain: A Mattress Misstep

Early in my career with Slight Motion PT, I was blindsided by a nagging hip pain. According to this MRI, I have a torn labrum in both hips and could've easily blamed that for my struggles. As a physical therapist, I knew the exercises, the stretches, the techniques—and I practiced them religiously. But week after week, the ache lingered, creeping in with an almost mocking persistence. I started to wonder if something else might be triggering the pain.

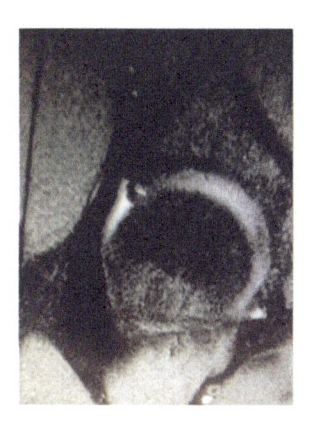

Then, in a flash, it came to me: the mattress.

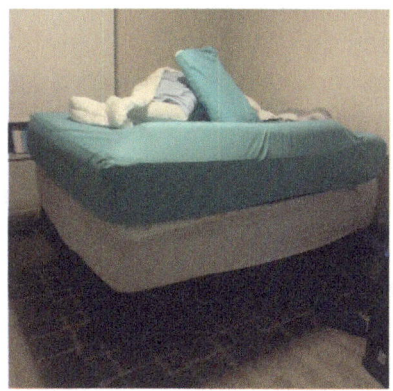

Not that I'm saying mattresses are typically the problem—more often than not, it's something we're doing.

But in my case, I realized I had a unique issue with my mattress. I had a smart mattress that adjusts its temperature to keep you comfortable through the night. Unfortunately, it had recently flooded, and while the company promptly sent me a replacement, there was a slight hiccup in my setup. Unable to move the old mattress out of my room alone, I stacked the two mattresses temporarily.

Every night, this setup forced me into an acrobatic event:

I'd back up, take a little running start, jump slightly, and swing my leg over the elevated surface- all just to get into bed. It became such a routine that I stopped thinking about it. Just another part of my day, like brushing my teeth or checking my phone. Then one day, it hit me. My hip pain had started right around the time of the mattress flood. Could my nightly gymnastics routine be the culprit? This minor but repetitive maneuver was putting unexpected strain on my hip. Once I made the connection, I immediately asked a neighbor for help to haul the old mattress out. That night, with just one mattress in place, I climbed into bed normally. It was as if my hip was relieved. Within days, the persistent ache began to fade. It wasn't about needing more exercises or better stretches, I was already doing everything else correctly. It was about stopping the nightly movement that was irritating my hip.

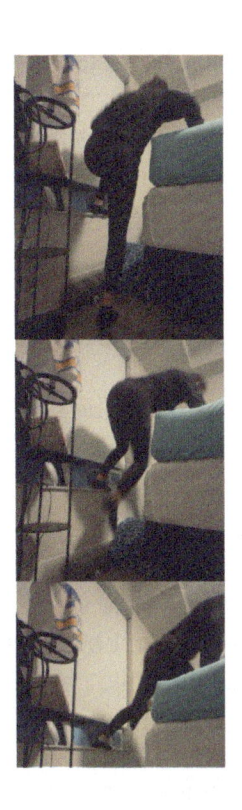

This experience taught me something profound: sometimes the smallest details in our routine can create surprisingly big consequences for how we feel. We often overlook the everyday movements and patterns that shape our body's comfort. It made me wonder: could something as simple as getting in and out of bed be affecting others' hip health too?

Take a "routine audit" of your day:

- What movements do you do without thinking?
- How do you get in and out of bed?
- What "temporary" adaptations have become permanent?
- What solutions might be creating new problems?

This realization changed how I approach patient care. It reminded me that while we often look for complex solutions to pain, sometimes the answer is hiding in the simple movements we do every day. As I tell my clients now, "The things we do without thinking often affect us more than the things we do with intention."

Small Changes, Big Results

Hip pain often originates from the small, everyday actions and habits that we don't even realize are contributing to discomfort. By becoming more aware of how we move, sit, and sleep, we can make simple adjustments that have a profound impact on our health. Whether it's repositioning your workspace, adjusting your sleep posture, or changing the way you get in and out of bed, these small shifts can lead to big improvements in hip health and overall well-being.

The key to managing and preventing hip pain lies in tuning into your body's needs. By addressing the root causes—often hidden within the routines we take for granted—you can reduce discomfort, increase stability, and improve your quality of life.

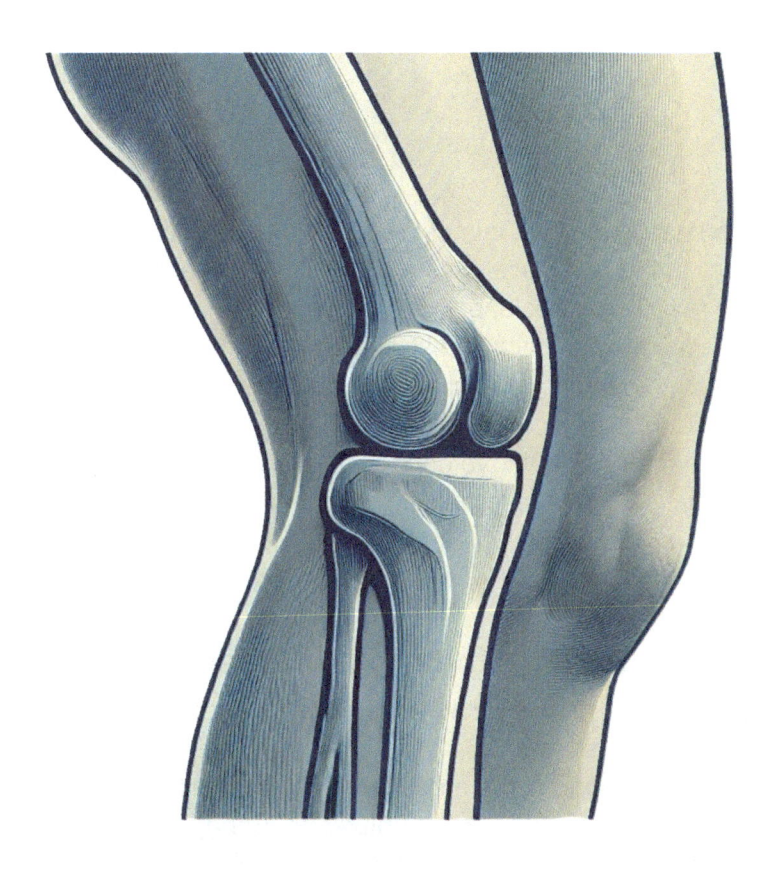

Chapter 10
Knee Knowledge

Knee Knowledge

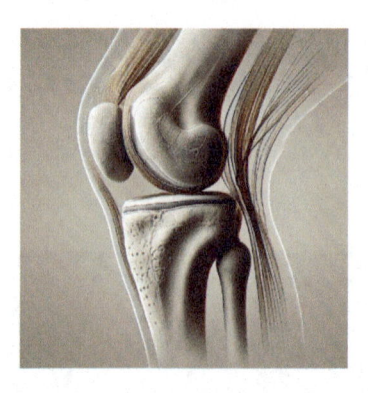

The knee is one of the most remarkable yet vulnerable joints in the body, acting as a critical link between your hips and feet. It absorbs shock, stabilizes movement, and provides the flexibility and strength needed for walking, running, squatting, and climbing. However, its constant use and complex structure make it prone to injury and degeneration, leading to conditions like ligament tears, meniscus injuries, and patellar pain. In this chapter, we'll provide practical insights to keep this vital joint strong, stable, and pain-free for years to come.

Understanding Knee Pain: Causes, Solutions, and Prevention

Knee pain is one of the most common complaints among individuals of all ages, from athletes to grandparents, in fact it is one of the most common reasons for visits to orthopedic surgeons. According to the American Academy of Orthopaedic Surgeons (AAOS), nearly 1 in 4 adults suffer from chronic knee pain.[17]

THE "A" WORD

Arthritis – have you been told you have arthritis or "bone on bone"?

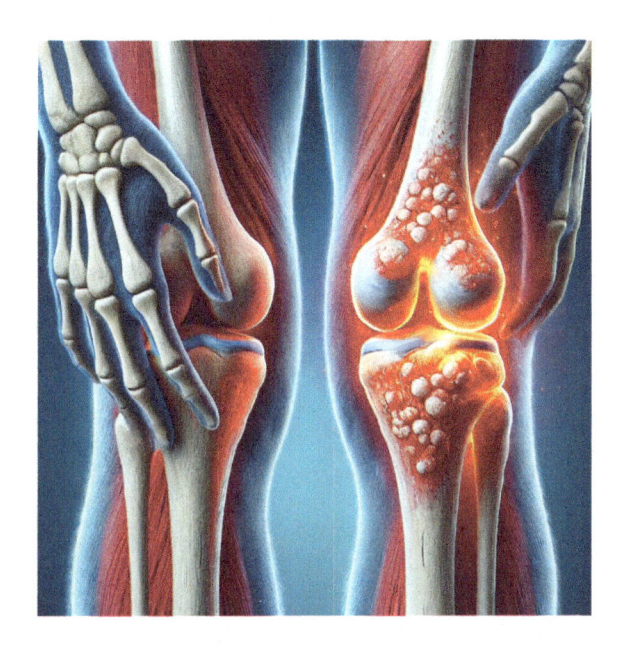

If you've been told that arthritis is the cause of your knee pain, you're not alone. Arthritis is often blamed for knee pain, but did you know that many people with visible signs of arthritis on MRIs don't even experience pain?

Studies show that around 19-43% of people over age 40 have knee arthritis without symptoms[18]. Another study reported that nearly all knees (97%) of asymptomatic adults showed abnormalities in at least one knee structure on MRI[19].

Don't let a diagnosis of arthritis make you feel like surgery is inevitable—there are conservative options that can provide significant relief.

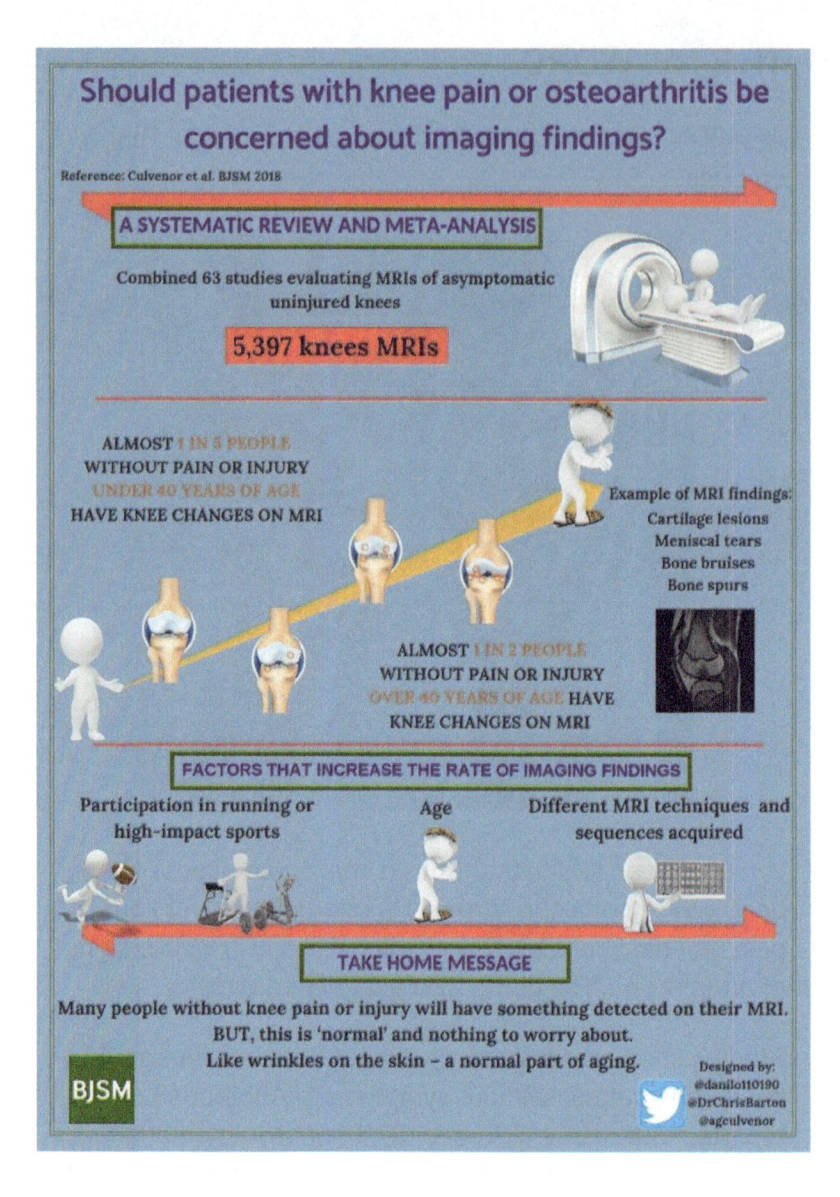

MRI findings in asymptomatic individuals. Designed by @danilo110190, Dr. Chris Barton, and A.G. Culvenor. Data from Culvenor, A. G., et al. (2018). *British Journal of Sports Medicine*, 53(20), 1265–1275. doi:10.1136/bjsports-2018-099257.

Kneeling: A Hidden Cause of Knee Pain

Kneeling is a common activity, whether for cleaning, gardening, or even playing with children, but it can be a significant source of knee pain. Many of my clients have come to me with fluctuating knee pain, and through careful analysis, we've discovered that the simplest activities, like kneeling, are often the culprits. Think about the load and weight going directly through the knee. It is not meant to bear your full weight. With a few of the clients, we came to the conclusion that it was their kneeling to clean the floor that triggered their pain. When they stopped kneeling their knee pain went away.

One client had knee pain that seemed to come and go without any clear cause. During a session, she casually mentioned cleaning out her kitchen cabinets and gave me a jar of jam as a thank-you gift. This prompted me to ask her to demonstrate how she cleaned her cabinets. She kneeled on the floor, took everything out, and then put it back in. When I asked how often she did this, she replied, "Every two weeks."

This routine was a clear trigger for her knee pain. The pain would start a couple of days after cleaning, last for about a week, and just as it began to subside, she would start the cycle again by cleaning her cabinets. This pattern is common—many people don't realize that their knee pain is caused by activities that seem harmless but are performed in ways that strain the knee joint.

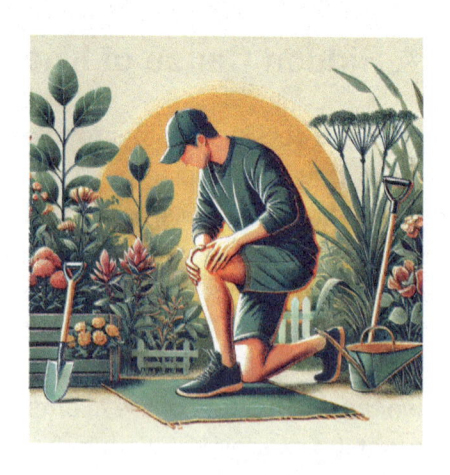

Gardening is another activity that often involves kneeling, and it's a frequent source of knee pain for my clients. One client mentioned that his knee had started giving out randomly, something that hadn't happened in a long time. As we discussed his recent activities, he mentioned that he had been gardening more frequently because of the warmer weather.

When I asked if he knelt while gardening, he confirmed that he did, and the pain had started the day after a long gardening session. This realization was a breakthrough for him—he hadn't connected the dots between his kneeling and his knee pain.

Kneeling, especially on hard surfaces, puts significant pressure on the kneecap, underlying cartilage, and the soft tissues surrounding the knee joint. Over time, this pressure can lead to inflammation, pain, and even long-term cartilage damage. The *Journal of Orthopaedic & Sports Physical Therapy* reports that prolonged kneeling, particularly on hard surfaces, is a risk factor for developing knee pain and conditions like prepatellar bursitis.[20]

I have personal experience with the effects of kneeling on knee pain. I randomly started getting knee pain and originally just blamed it on the cartilage damage I have. If a client didn't have a chair for me to sit on while I worked on their neck I would kneel. I realized I would have minor to moderate discomfort a few days later. Despite my best efforts to manage the pain through exercises and stretches and decrease my kneeling time, it persisted. I realized that even short periods of only 3 minutes of kneeling were enough to trigger my knee pain, likely due to my history of patella dislocations and cartilage damage. I personally can't even kneel on pews without having residual pain a few days later. If I had continued to kneel regularly without addressing the underlying issue, the pain could have compounded, leading me to believe I might need an MRI or even another surgery. This experience taught me the importance of avoiding unnecessary kneeling and being mindful of the strain we place on our knees during everyday activities.

Knee Pain and Stomach Sleeping: An Overlooked Connection

Another surprising contributor to knee pain is stomach sleeping. This position can put pressure on the kneecap, particularly if the knee is pressed into the mattress or if the leg is extended in a way that strains the joint. After my patella dislocations, I couldn't lay on my stomach for an extended period without experiencing discomfort in my knees. A study published in Clinical Orthopaedics and Related Research found that certain sleep positions, including stomach sleeping, can exacerbate existing knee pain or even contribute to the development of pain over time.[21]

As discussed in our Pillow Talk chapter, we know stomach sleeping is the worst position to sleep in for many reasons and you should try to implement the Four Pillow Method to transition to side sleeping.

Do You Know How Much Pressure Your Knees Endure?

When you stand still, your knees bear 80% of your body weight, and when you walk, they take on 150% or more. That means losing even one pound of body weight results in a 4 pound reduction in the pressure on your knees. Losing just 10 pounds would relieve 40 pounds of pressure from your knees, significantly reducing the strain on your joints. Consider using an ergonomic mat to reduce the load on your knees if you're standing for long periods.

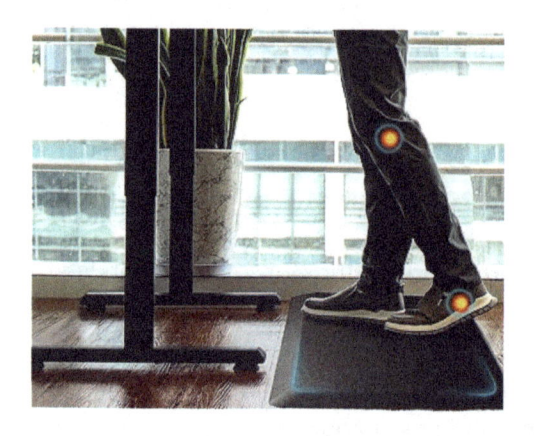

The Benefits of Kinesiotaping for Knee Pain

Kinesiotaping is a technique that I've found particularly helpful in managing knee pain, both for myself and my clients. Kinesiotape can help reduce pain by providing support, improving circulation, and decreasing pressure on the affected area.

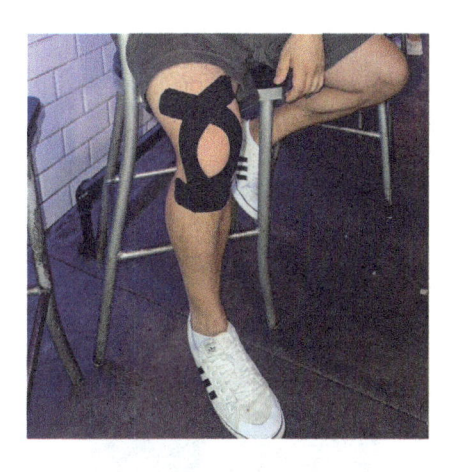

I recall a time when I experienced severe knee pain, which caused my knee to lock, making it difficult to walk. I was concerned that I might need another surgery, as a locked knee can indicate a loose body or "catching" of the meniscus in the joint, which typically requires surgical intervention. At the time I could only walk with my foot extremely externally rotated like a duck. However, my professor Dr. David Capote, who teaches Kinematic Taping courses, applied a rotational offload taping technique, which immediately relieved the pressure, and my knee unlocked. Since then, I haven't experienced any locking.

Kinesiotaping can also be a valuable alternative to surgery in some cases. I saw that a friend of mine on Instagram was diagnosed with a meniscus tear and she was convinced that she needed surgery. When she was asking for surgeon recommendations, I pitched her on at least letting me try taping it first before going under the knife. After applying the tape, she felt almost immediate relief and was able to manage her condition with physical therapy, ultimately avoiding surgery. This situation has happened multiple times since then and I've been able to get a lot of people to cancel surgery by almost instantly taking away their pain.

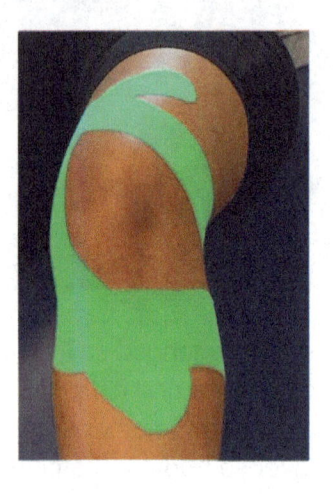

Most people have some type of damage under the kneecap. It's like the tires on your car having some type of wear and tear. When it gets irritated, the knee cap can start moving in an improper groove and increase irritation, inflammation, and pain. I think the tape is so beneficial because it helps offload that area and surrounding structures to give the knee some relief from the constant exacerbation.

However, not everyone in the medical field is supportive of taping. I once met an Orthopedic Surgeon who expressed frustration when patients came in with tape on their knees because it interfered with his ability to administer injections. This raises an important question: why are we so quick to resort to injections or surgery when less invasive options like taping can provide significant relief?

My Journey With Knee Surgery

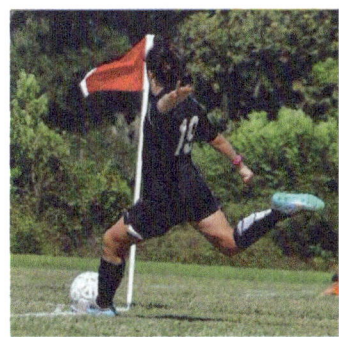

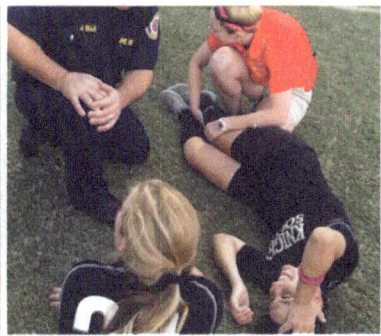

I have a history of knee pain dating back to high school soccer. I played on two of the top teams in the nation where we won a few state titles. I vividly remember the day I hurt my knee for the first time. We were practicing on a worn down practice field so we could finish early and the Coach said "No one better get hurt". I decided to shoot as hard as I could for fun and when I landed nothing absorbed the shock and it went straight to my knee. I immediately went down and knew I was injured. Something was wrong. I battled this injury for the next 6 months with rehab, but I NEVER did my home exercises because they wanted me to lay down and lift my leg, how boring. The exercises just seemed tedious and there were too many.

My knee would randomly click and lock for days where I'd be unable to walk. The discomfort was so bad that I remember I would promise myself if it went away it wouldn't be worth it to play soccer again. It would go away and feel perfect and I would return to soccer happily, forgetting how much pain it caused me.

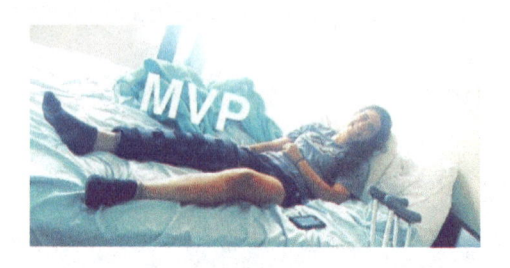

I ended up having to have surgery to remove a loose body that was getting caught and causing my knee to lock. I went to the best surgeon in town. It was this moment I realized I no longer wanted to be an Orthopedic Surgeon. The surgeon hardly even talked to me, he didn't care about me, I was just a patient. I wanted to be part of the recovery and I wanted to make the exercises so easy everyone would do them, and here we are.

A Pillow Gone Wrong

Speaking of knee surgery, one of the most important things they don't tell you after knee surgery is to NEVER put a pillow under your knee. Although it may feel more comfortable, this one pillow can be detrimental to your recovery.

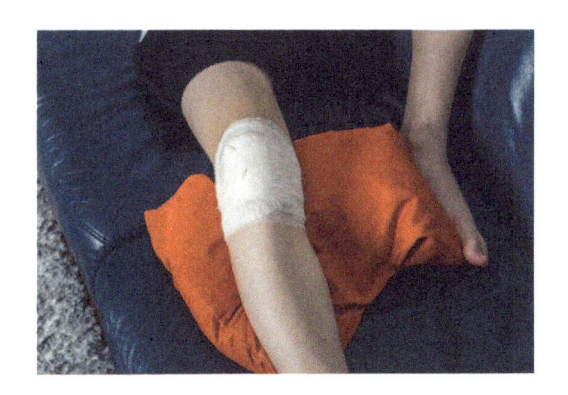

After her knee surgery, Karen was determined to heal quickly. Her surgeon had repaired a torn meniscus, and she left the hospital with detailed instructions for recovery: rest, ice, elevate, and gradually regain movement. Wanting to stay as comfortable as possible, Karen propped a soft pillow under her knee every time she sat or lay down. It felt soothing, relieving the tension around her joint. It became routine—her constant companion through naps, TV marathons, and even bedtime.

Weeks passed, and she grew frustrated. Despite following her rehab exercises diligently, her knee didn't feel right. Standing felt stiff, walking had turned into limping, and fully straightening her leg seemed impossible. During our session I watched her limp around the house like a pirate. Her knee stayed slightly bent when she walked, during the midstance phase when most of the weight is being transferred through the leg.

After testing her knee's range of motion, I asked, "Do you sleep or rest with a pillow under your knee?"

She nodded. "It's the only way I feel comfortable."

"That's part of the problem," I explained. "The pillow might feel good now, but it's keeping your knee stuck in a bent position. Your body is learning to stay there. If we don't address this, it'll impact how you walk, how your muscles work, and even your recovery long-term."

Karen was stunned. She had no idea that something as simple as a pillow could hinder her healing. I explained further: "When your knee stays bent for too long, your hamstrings stay tight, and your quadriceps aren't able to engage properly. This prevents your leg from fully straightening, which you need for normal walking. Without full extension, your gait mechanics shift, and the rest of your body compensates—leading to limping, muscle imbalances, and even more pain from this lack of range of motion"

I encouraged Karen to stop using the knee pillow and to focus on the exercises to regain full extension. It wasn't easy at first. Karen missed the comfort of her pillow and felt the tension as her knee adjusted to its new, straighter position. But within a few days, things started to change. She stood taller, felt steadier, and the limp she'd grown accustomed to began to fade.

Two weeks later, she walked into our next session with a noticeable difference. Her gait was smooth, her leg extended fully with every step, and no limping!

"It's incredible," Karen said. "Who knew a pillow could hold me back so much?"

I nodded. "Sometimes the smallest habits can have the biggest impact. Getting rid of that pillow gave your knee the space to heal and move the way it's supposed to. Full extension is key to everything—walking, running, and living pain-free. It may not seem like much, but even just a few degrees makes the biggest difference in your walking mechanics"

From then on, Karen's pillow stayed where it belonged: on her bed, under her head, and far away from her knee.

Another piece of advice I like to give my clients post surgery is the 1 minute-every-hour rule. If you move your joint for one hour a day at PT or do a few exercises in 5 minutes, then the other 23 hours the knee will be stiff. We should be going through a tolerable full range of motion for 1 minute every hour to keep the muscles and joint looser.

Knee Pain and Desk Posture: A Common Overlooked Cause

Do you have anything hiding under your desk? Possibly something you like to rest your feet on while on the phone or during zoom meetings?

Desk posture is a significant yet often overlooked contributor to knee pain. Many people spend hours sitting at desks with poor posture, which can strain the knees, especially if the workspace is not ergonomically designed.

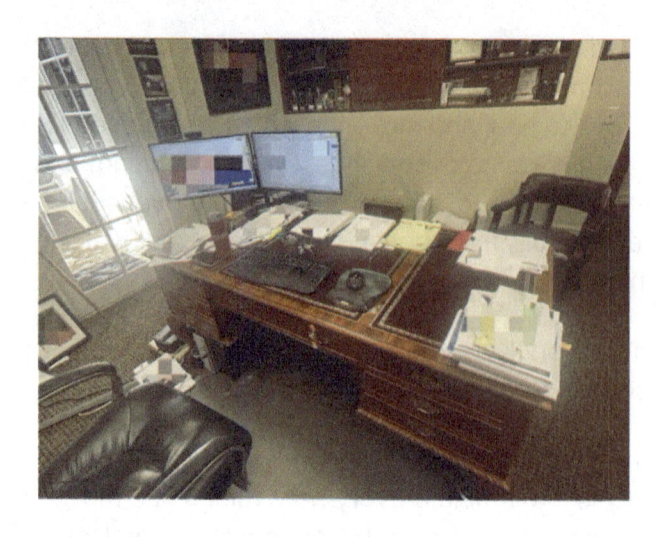

One of my clients came to me with pain in his right knee, specifically in the lateral collateral ligament (LCL), which runs along the outside of the knee. This pain was particularly noticeable when he performed lunges to the right. After visiting his office, I noticed that his monitor was positioned far to the left, forcing him to twist his body and strain his right knee throughout the day. Additionally, he had a small cubby under his desk where he rested his legs, further exacerbating the issue by restricting his leg movements.

This setup was putting continuous stress on his LCL, leading to pain. Once we adjusted his workspace, centering his monitor and replacing the desk, his knee pain began to improve. This case highlights the importance of proper desk ergonomics in preventing knee pain.

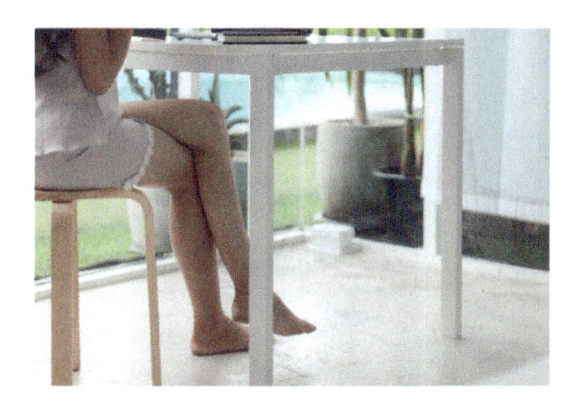

Criss-crossing the legs while sitting, another common habit, can also stress the ligaments in the knees, leading to discomfort. It is often found that sitting with legs crossed for extended periods can increase the risk of knee pain by creating uneven pressure on the joints and stretching the ligaments which are meant to be tight to prevent collapse and excess stress.

Avoiding Knee Pain at the Gym: The Leg Extension Machine and Lunges

Knee pain can also be exacerbated by certain exercises, particularly when performed incorrectly. One exercise that often causes knee issues is the leg extension machine. This machine isolates the quadriceps, putting a significant load on the knee joint, especially when used with heavy weights. It's not always an exercise that should be avoided, but there are right and wrong ways to perform it, especially when having your knee's best interest in mind.

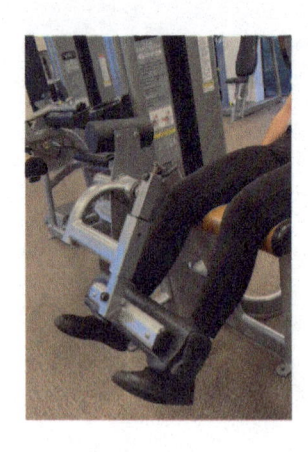

I had a client who regularly used the leg extension machine with over 100 pounds of weight, performing single-leg extensions. She began experiencing knee pain, which subsided after she reduced the load. While the leg extension machine can be beneficial for strengthening the quadriceps, overloading it can place excessive stress on the knee, particularly the patellar tendon, leading to pain. Over and over again I've been able to solve and decrease knee pain by having the client pick alternative exercises to the leg extension machine, which places undue stress on the average person's knee.

Are You Performing Lunges Correctly?

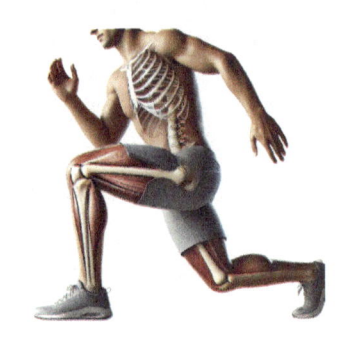

Lunges are another exercise that, if performed incorrectly, can cause knee pain. When lunging, it's important to ensure that the knee tracks toward the outside of the big toe rather than caving inward. A knee that caves inward places excessive stress on the medial compartment of the knee, increasing the risk of injury. This is called "knee valgus". The amount of people I watch in the gym performing lunges toward the big toe is unreal, it makes me cringe.

A study published in the *Journal of Orthopaedic & Sports Physical Therapy* emphasizes the importance of proper form during exercises like lunges to avoid undue stress on the knee joint. Strengthening the glutes and core can help your body to naturally maintain proper alignment during these movements, reducing the risk of knee pain.

Patellar Maltracking: Understanding and Addressing the Issue

Patellar maltracking occurs when the kneecap (patella) does not move properly within its groove during knee movements. This condition is a common cause of anterior knee pain and can lead to conditions like patellofemoral pain syndrome (PFPS) or chondromalacia patellae, where the cartilage under the kneecap becomes damaged.

Patellar maltracking often results from muscle imbalances, particularly weakness in the quadriceps, hip abductors, and glutes. It can also be exacerbated by improper foot positioning during activities like lunging or stepping abruptly to the side.

Correcting patellar maltracking involves strengthening the muscles that support proper knee alignment and avoiding activities that place excessive stress on the knee joint.

Banded exercises to engage the glutes, such as *side steps* or *clamshells*, can help improve muscle balance and reduce the risk of patellar maltracking.

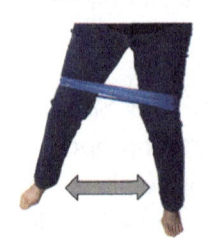

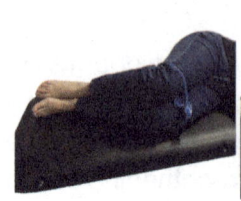

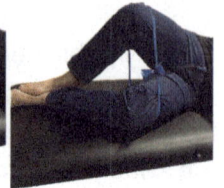

What Small Changes Can You Make to Alleviate Knee Pain?

Knee pain is often caused by the small, everyday habits we don't even realize are harmful. Adjusting how you kneel, sit, and workout can have a huge impact. Whether it's modifying your desk setup, sleeping position, or exercise routine, simple changes can lead to big improvements in your knee health. The **Slight Motion Method** can help identify and correct these habits before they lead to more serious issues. Movement is medicine, and small, consistent adjustments can provide long-term relief.

Chapter 11
Footwork
Fundamentals

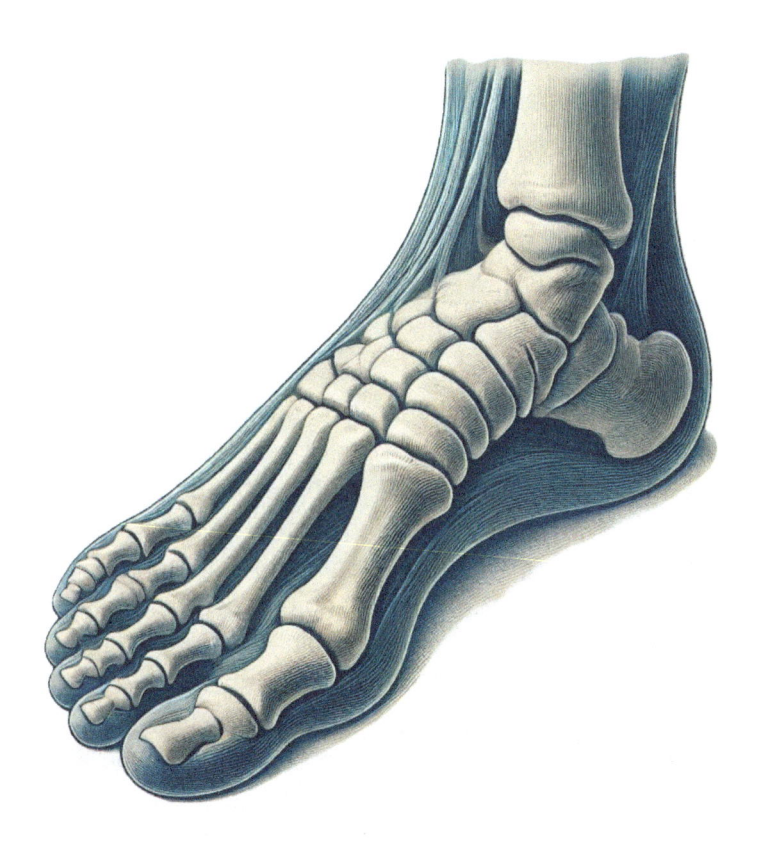

Footwork Fundamentals

The foot and ankle are the foundation of your body, supporting every step you take and absorbing the forces of daily movement. However, this foundation is often overlooked until pain or dysfunction sets in. In our experience, some of the most common diagnoses involving the foot and ankle we see are plantar fasciitis, achilles tendinitis, ankle sprains, and issues related to flat feet or high arches. These conditions can disrupt walking, balance, and posture, leading to compensations elsewhere in the body. This chapter explores the essential role of foot and ankle health, the habits that contribute to these problems, and the fundamental strategies to restore strength, mobility, and stability—ensuring every step is a step in the right direction.

Plantar fasciitis is one of the most common causes of heel pain, resulting from inflammation of the plantar fascia—a thick band of tissue that runs along the bottom of your foot, connecting your heel bone to your toes. This tissue acts like a shock absorber, supporting the arch of your foot during walking and standing. When overused or strained, the plantar fascia can develop small tears, leading to irritation and pain. It's typically felt as a sharp or stabbing sensation near the heel, especially with the first steps in the morning or after prolonged periods of inactivity, like sitting. Factors like improper footwear, sleep positions, tight calf muscle, or abnormal foot mechanics often contribute to this condition.

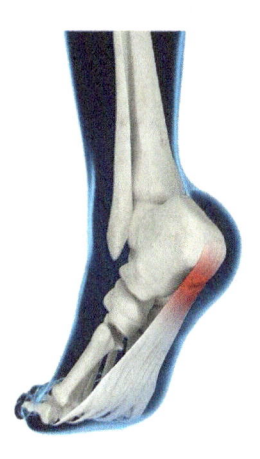

Alyssa's Battle with Plantar Fasciitis

Alyssa, a 42-year-old marketing executive, came to me with debilitating heel pain that had plagued her for months. "I can barely get out of bed in the morning," she admitted. Desperate for relief, she had tried every tip she found on the internet: icing, stretching, and expensive orthotics, but nothing worked.

"I thought I was doing everything right," she said, frustrated.

But here's the issue—what we often hear or read about plantar fasciitis doesn't always align with what we should actually be doing. Plantar fasciitis is caused by a lack of blood flow to the plantar fascia, leading to tissue irritation and microtears. While icing is commonly recommended, it actually reduces blood flow even further, which delays healing. Instead, we need to focus on increasing circulation to the area.

I suggested Alyssa switch from icing to heat therapy. Something as simple as closing the drain during her shower to let warm water pool around her feet, or soaking them in a warm bowl with Epsom salt, can improve circulation and help relieve her pain. I also mentioned that contrast baths—alternating between warm and cold water—might provide relief.

Another common misconception is that stretching helps. For Alyssa, the advice to stretch her plantar fascia was actually making things worse by pulling on the already irritated tissue. Instead, I recommended giving her fascia a break by doing the opposite of stretching—scrunching her toes downward toward her heel to contract the tissue and increase blood flow to promote healing.

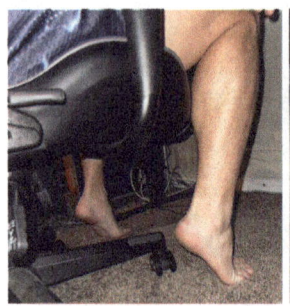

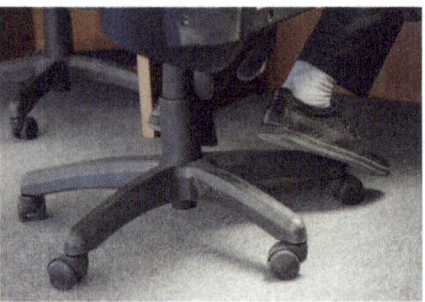

When we examined her daily habits, the root of her pain became even clearer. At her desk, Alyssa rarely kept her feet flat on the floor. She often rested her heels on the legs of her chair or held them slightly elevated in a calf-raise-like position.

This constant shortening of the calf muscles created tightness that fueled her plantar fasciitis. On top of that, she was a stomach sleeper, which kept her ankles in plantarflexion all night, further tightening her calves and placing stress on the plantar fascia.

The solution was simple but effective:
- **Desk Ergonomics**: I had Alyssa adjust her workstation to ensure her feet rested flat on the floor. We added a small footrest for support and encouraged her to roll a tennis ball under her foot periodically to relieve tension.
- **Sleep Adjustments**: I suggested she try side sleeping to reduce strain on her plantar fascia. As a temporary solution, she could also hang her feet off the edge of the bed to maintain a neutral ankle position.
- **Heat Therapy**: Soaking her feet in warm water or using a contrast bath became part of her evening routine.

Within a few weeks, Alyssa reported significant improvements. "The morning pain is almost gone," she said, relieved. "I had no idea how much my desk setup and sleep habits were affecting me."

Key Takeaways

- **Rethink Icing and Stretching:** Icing reduces blood flow, which plantar fascia needs to heal. Instead, consider heat therapy to improve circulation, and avoid stretching the fascia—focus on scrunching the toes to instead shorten the tissue and promote healing.
- **Daily Habits Matter:** Almost every client I treat with plantar fasciitis sits with their heels off the ground and sleeps on their stomach. Both habits lead to tight calves and strain on the fascia.

Plantar fasciitis is rarely caused by a single factor, but by addressing these subtle, daily habits, you can avoid unnecessary pain and find the relief you've been searching for.

Emily's Secret to Calf Strength

Emily, a 29-year-old marathon runner, came to me with recurring calf pain that was holding her back during training. "I feel like my calves are constantly fatigued," she said. "By the end of my long runs, I can barely keep going." Emily had always focused on building endurance, but she hadn't considered the importance of targeted calf strengthening.

When I assessed her, it became clear that her calves were underprepared for the demands of marathon running. While the calves may seem like a small, unimportant muscle group, they perform a huge job. They generate more force than even the glutes and thighs during running. According to *Runner's World*, the quadriceps operate at around 63% of their maximum capacity while running, with the calves potentially enduring even greater strain—up to 84% of their maximum strength during each stride.[22] This makes calf strength a critical factor for endurance athletes like Emily.

Physiotherapist Alison Rose emphasizes that "good calf strength is my number one non-negotiable requirement for runners." According to Rose, runners should be able to perform three sets of 25 single-leg calf raises with both a bent knee and a straight knee at the end of a run. Each rep should go to full range, and there should be no shaking or wobbling during the movement.

Emily had never performed a dedicated calf-strengthening routine, and her lack of preparation showed. "I can barely do 10 single-leg raises," she admitted after a quick test. Together, we developed a plan to build her calf strength gradually, focusing on:

Straight-Knee Raises: Targeting the gastrocnemius muscle.

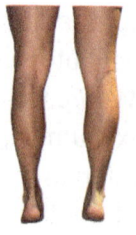

Bent-Knee Raises: Engaging the soleus muscle, essential for supporting endurance activities.

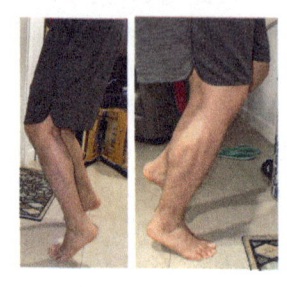

We started with two sets of 15 reps per leg, progressively increasing to three sets of 25. I also encouraged Emily to incorporate her calf routine into her post-run cooldown when her muscles were already fatigued, mimicking the conditions they'd face during a race.

The Results

Three weeks later, Emily came back stronger—and faster. "I ran 18 miles last weekend without any calf pain," she said, beaming. Not only had her pain disappeared, but she also felt more stable and efficient during her runs. "I can feel my calves carrying me through the tougher stretches," she added.

Key Takeaway

- Calf Strength is Critical for Runners: The calves are responsible for a disproportionately high amount of force during running—84% of their maximum capability compared to 63% for the quads.
- Strength Benchmarks: Runners should self test and aim for three sets of 25 single-leg calf raises (both bent and straight knees), going to full range without wobbling.
- Build Strength Under Fatigue: Incorporate calf exercises into your post-run cooldown to simulate race conditions and build resilience.

For marathon runners, the calves are the unsung heroes, driving speed, endurance, and reducing the risk of injury.

The Overlooked Soleus: The Missing Piece in Achilles Injury Prevention

When it comes to preventing and recovering from Achilles tendon injuries, the soleus muscle is often overlooked. Sitting beneath the larger, more visible calf muscle, the soleus plays a critical role in supporting the Achilles tendon and absorbing forces during walking, running, and jumping. Unlike the calf, which is primarily active during explosive movements when the knee is straight, the soleus works hardest when the knee is bent. This subtle difference is key—many training programs fail to isolate and strengthen the soleus effectively, leaving the Achilles tendon a prime suspect for injury.

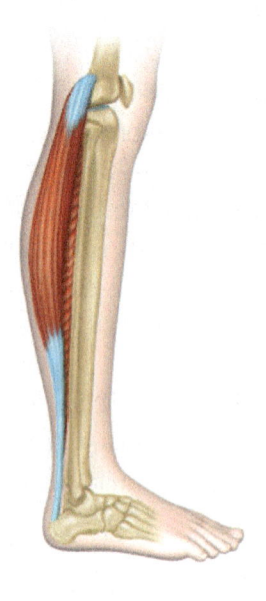

The soleus acts as a shock absorber, bearing up to 8 times your body weight during activities like running and jumping. If the soleus is weak or undertrained, the Achilles tendon is forced to take on more load, increasing the risk of overuse injuries like Achilles tendinitis or even ruptures. Targeted exercises, such as bent-knee calf raises and eccentric training help build strength and endurance in this deep muscle.

Neglecting the soleus is like ignoring the foundation of a building—it might hold up for a while, but under repetitive stress, cracks begin to appear. Incorporating focused soleus training into your routine can be the missing piece to reducing Achilles strain, improving resilience, and keeping your movements pain-free and powerful.

The Case of Ken and the Mysterious Calf Pain

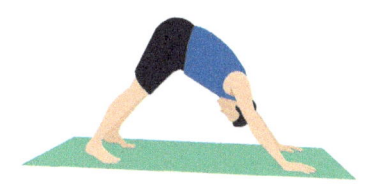

Ken, a 55-year-old yoga enthusiast, came to me with calf pain so persistent it was beginning to interfere with his downward dog pose. "I've stretched, foam rolled, and even tried acupuncture," he told me in frustration. "Nothing works." His doctors had shrugged it off as a normal part of aging, but something about his story didn't add up.

When I asked about his daily habits, he mentioned working from home at a desk. Curious, I decided to do a home assessment. As we walked into his workspace, the culprit became clear: a stack of weights tucked neatly under his desk.

"What's this?" I asked. "Oh, I rest my feet on them sometimes," Ken said, shrugging. "It's just comfortable."

But this small habit was putting his calves in a stretched, downward angle for hours every day. The constant pull on his muscles was creating strain and dysfunction. It wasn't his yoga practice causing the pain—it was the way he sat.

The solution was simple: we removed the weights, adjusted his desk setup, and added a few exercises like single-leg calf raises and dynamic stretches to mobilize the tissue. Within a week, Ken's pain started to subside. By the end of the month, he was back to yoga, pain-free.

"I never realized something so small could have such a big impact," he said.

Key Takeaway

Small daily habits—like resting your feet on an uneven surface—can create unnecessary strain on your calves. Check your workspace for hidden culprits that might be affecting your posture and muscle health.

Jenny's Journey to Toe Independence

Jenny, a 34-year-old runner, complained of persistent foot pain during long-distance training. After a quick assessment, I noticed she couldn't lift her big toe independently—a sign of poor foot control and weak arch support.

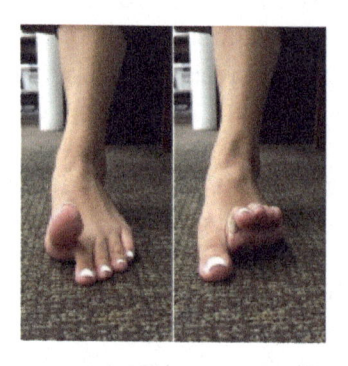

We introduced toe mobility drills, like lifting the big toe while keeping the others down, and vice versa. Toe spacers helped realign her foot mechanics. Within a month, her arch strength improved, and her pain diminished. "It's amazing how something so small can make such a difference," she said.

The Shoe Switch That Saved Diane's Ankle

Diane was an avid walker who loved her daily 5-mile treks. But recently, she'd been experiencing persistent ankle pain. An orthopedic surgeon recommended surgery, citing ligament laxity as the cause. But something didn't add up. Diane's ankle let her walk five miles a day—why would it suddenly require surgery?

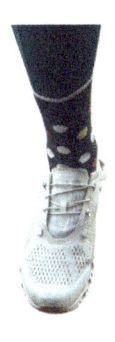

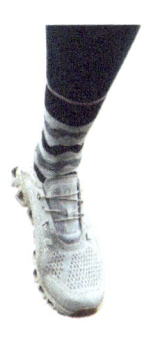

In our first session I noticed Diane was wearing bungee-laced shoes. "These are so easy," she said, demonstrating how she slid them on without untying them. That convenience was the problem. Without proper tension from the laces, her foot was sliding inside the shoe, forcing her ankle to overwork for stability.

Coincidentally, that same week, I had developed lateral ankle pain after switching to a pair of these bungee-laced shoes myself. Additionally, two clients reported similar ankle pain that week, which they attributed to their history of ankle sprains. Both were also wearing the same bungee-laced shoes. Upon further investigation, I realized the shoes were likely contributing to the problem.

I recommended switching to supportive lace-up shoes and tying them every time she put them on. Within days, Diane noticed a difference. After a month, her ankle pain was gone. Surgery? Unnecessary. "I'll never buy shoes without proper laces again," she laughed.

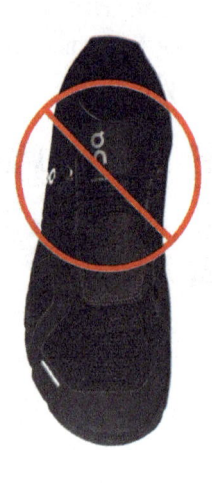

Key Takeaway

Properly tied, supportive shoes are essential for foot and ankle health. Don't sacrifice function for convenience.

- Shoes Can Make or Break Your Ankle Health: Slip-on or bungee-laced shoes might be convenient, but they often lack the stability needed to support your foot during activity, leading to unnecessary strain on the ankle.
- Proper Lacing is Essential: Always tie your shoes snugly before exercising or walking to ensure your foot remains stable inside the shoe.
- Avoid Unnecessary Interventions: Small changes, like switching shoes and incorporating ankle-strengthening exercises, can often prevent more invasive treatments, like surgery!

Sometimes the solution to chronic pain isn't as complicated as it seems. Diane's story is a reminder that the right footwear—and the simple act of tying your laces—can go a long way in keeping you pain-free and active.

Mark and the Calf Cramp Mystery

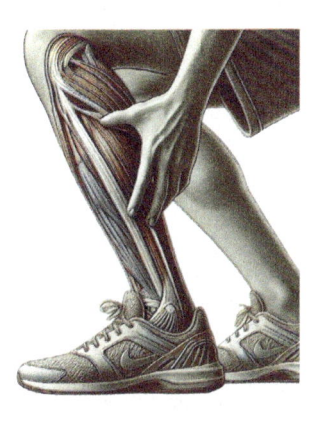

Mark, a 38-year-old tech consultant, came to me with recurring calf cramps and stiffness. He'd tried magnesium supplements, massages, and stretching routines, but nothing seemed to help. "It just hits me out of nowhere," he said.

When I asked about his hydration habits, Mark sheepishly admitted to drinking only 16 ounces of water a day—"I drink a lot of coffee," he added. That was the problem. His muscles were screaming for hydration, and coffee's diuretic effects were only making it worse.

I challenged Mark to double his water to coffee intake. We also added simple calf-strengthening exercises, like single-leg calf raises, to build resilience. Within two weeks, Mark's cramps disappeared. "I feel like a new person, it hasn't happened since!" he said.

Key Takeaway

Hydration is key to muscle health. If you're experiencing cramps, start by increasing your water intake before looking for more complicated solutions.

Linda's Summer Sandal Problem

Linda, a 49-year-old avid traveler, came to me with a familiar complaint: "Every summer, my feet ache, and my ankles swell, especially after walking a lot on vacation. It doesn't happen in winter, though." When I asked about her footwear, Linda sheepishly admitted, "I love flip-flops. They're just so easy."

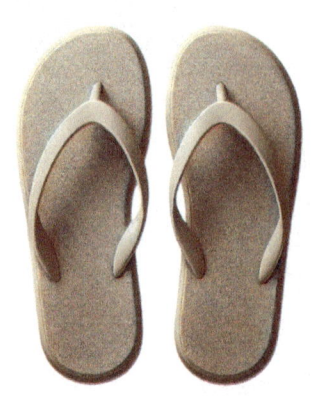

Flip-flops offer almost no support, forcing the foot's tendons and muscles to grip constantly to keep the shoe in place. On uneven surfaces, this lack of support strains the arch, ankle, ligaments, and calf muscle. Linda's vacation habits, exploring cobblestone streets and walking long distances, were exacerbating the issue.

I recommended supportive walking shoes for sightseeing and suggested wearing flip-flops only sparingly, like at the beach. We also introduced foot-strengthening exercises, like toe scrunches and towel pickups, to rebuild her foot stability.

Two months later, Linda emailed me a photo of her walking confidently through Paris in proper shoes. "I thought I'd miss my flip-flops, but I don't miss the pain!" she wrote.

Barbara's "Arthritis" That Wasn't

Barbara, a 62-year-old grandmother, had been diagnosed with arthritis after months of ankle pain. She'd tried braces, medication, and injections, but the pain persisted. "I've accepted this is just part of aging," she told me during our initial consultation. But as she described her daily life, one detail caught my attention.

Barbara often wore a particular pair of slip-on shoes for errands because they were "so easy to slide on." But when I tested her gait in those shoes, her foot wobbled with every step, forcing her ankle to compensate for the lack of stability. It wasn't arthritis—it was her shoe choice!

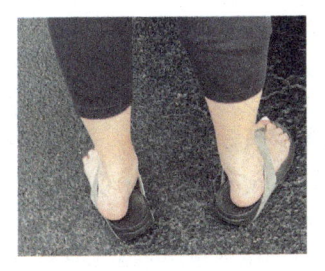

We replaced her slip-ons with a supportive pair of lace-up walking shoes. Within days, her pain improved.

With targeted exercises to strengthen her ankle and improve her balance, Barbara was back to gardening and playing with her grandkids within a month. "I can't believe it was that simple," she said.

The Curious Case of Nick's Ankle

Nick was a spirited 52-year-old who loved nothing more than attending outdoor music festivals with his family. But for the past two years, his post-event routine involved icing his swollen ankle and grimacing through the night. He chalked it up to the old soccer injury he had suffered years ago, but the discomfort was becoming more than an occasional inconvenience—it was limiting his life.

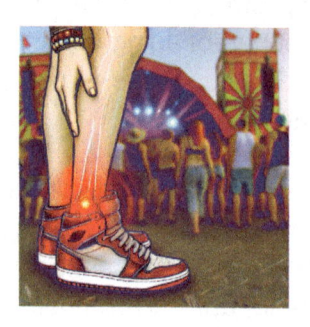

When Nick came to me, he mentioned that his ankle would start throbbing after walking for 30 minutes or standing in line at the store. He demonstrated a slight limp that he had subconsciously developed to "protect" his ankle, though it only made things worse.

To get to the root of the issue, I asked him to try a simple balance test: standing on one leg. He chuckled nervously but gave it a shot. Within five seconds, he stumbled. His other leg came down to catch him, and his eyes widened in disbelief.

"That's odd," he muttered, "I thought I had pretty good balance."

What I explained to Nick was simple yet revealing: If you can't balance on one leg for at least 30 seconds, your body is likely struggling to stabilize itself during everyday activities like walking, climbing stairs, or even standing still. Without that stability, the muscles and joints around the ankle are overworked, leading to the swelling and discomfort he had been dealing with for years.

Over the next few weeks, Nick committed to daily single-leg balance exercises. He started small—standing on one leg while brushing his teeth, holding onto the counter for extra stability. Gradually, we introduced more challenging moves: diagonal kickbacks, adding a slight turn of his head, and eventually balancing with his eyes closed.

One day, Nick came to a session with an unmistakable grin. "You're not gonna believe this," he said, "but last night, I kicked off my shoes without bracing myself against the wall. I haven't done that in years!"

Nick attended a weekend festival soon after and realized that his ankle didn't bother him at all. He stood for hours, walked for miles, and came home without needing the ice pack.

Like Nick, many people underestimate the power of balance in everyday movement. If you can't balance on one leg, your body compensates in ways that may cause pain or even lead to injuries and falls. Balance isn't just about staying upright—it's about enabling your body to move efficiently and maneuver uneven surfaces safely.

So, next time you're brushing your teeth, standing in line, or waiting for the microwave to ding, try standing on one leg. Can you make it to 30 seconds? How about with your eyes closed? As Nick's story shows, small changes, like improving your single-leg stability, can have a huge impact on reducing pain and restoring your freedom to move.

Your feet are the foundation of every step you take, bearing the weight of your body and propelling you forward through life. By understanding their mechanics and addressing common issues, you can improve balance, reduce pain, and enhance overall mobility. Small, consistent changes—like strengthening exercises, proper footwear choices, and mindful habits—can make a significant difference in how your feet function and feel. Remember, caring for your feet isn't just about comfort today; it's about creating a stable foundation for lifelong movement.

The Journey to a Pain-Free Life

As we come to the end of this book, it's clear that the little things truly matter. These stories aren't just things we've seen once. We included these specifically because it's the same habits contributing to similar pain we all experience. Each habit, each posture, each adjustment we make to our daily routines plays a role in shaping how we feel, move, and live. Pain, while complex and frustrating, is often the result of patterns we've unknowingly created over time. The good news is that the power to change those patterns lies in your hands.

At Slight Motion PT, our clients often tell us they've "tried everything" before finding us. Yet, after just one session using our proven Slight Motion Method, they experience significant improvements. We believe that awareness is key. By focusing on small, intentional changes, whether it's adjusting the way you sit, improving your sleep posture, or increasing how often you move, you can take powerful steps toward lasting comfort and mobility. With the Slight Motion Method, we don't just treat symptoms, we uncover and address the root causes of pain. It's the little changes that lead to big results, and we're here to help you make those changes today. Progress may feel slow at times, but remember, every little thing adds up. These small actions are like ripples that grow into waves, reshaping your relationship with your body and how it functions.

This book is not the end of your journey; it's the beginning of a lifelong commitment to mindful living and self-care. Celebrate the progress you've made, however small, and carry these lessons forward. Pain doesn't have to define your life—it's a signal, a teacher, and ultimately, an opportunity for growth.

Your body is resilient, capable of change and renewal. With awareness and effort, you can find relief, restore balance, and rediscover the joy of pain-free living. Keep moving forward, one small step at a time. After all, a little goes a long way…

References

1) Côté, P., Cassidy, J. D., & Carroll, L. (2008). The epidemiology of neck pain: What we have learned from our population-based studies. *Journal of Manipulative and Physiological Therapeutics, 31*(7), 459–464. Retrieved from https://pmc.ncbi.nlm.nih.gov/articles/PMC2974793/#:~:text=Neck%20pain%20is%20an%20important,to%20experience%20chronic%2C%20impairing%20pain
2) Myers, T. W. (2020). *Anatomy Trains: Myofascial Meridians for Manual and Movement Therapists* (4th ed.). Elsevier. Retrieved from https://www.anatomytrains.com.
3) Russell, B. S. (2008). "Carpal tunnel syndrome and the 'double crush' hypothesis: A review and implications for chiropractic." *Chiropractic & Osteopathy, 16*(2). doi:10.1186/1746-1340-16-2. Retrieved from https://pmc.ncbi.nlm.nih.gov/articles/PMC2365954/.
4) Hansraj, K. K. (2014). "Assessment of Stresses in the Cervical Spine Caused by Posture and Position of the Head." *Surgical Technology International*, 25, 277–279. Retrieved from https://surgicaltechnology.com.
5) Haugen, I. K., & Englund, M. (2019). "Hand Osteoarthritis — Clinical Features and Phenotypes." *Nature Reviews Rheumatology*, 15(11), 665–681. doi:10.1038/s41584-019-0319-y. Retrieved from https://doi.org/10.1038/s41584-019-0319-y.

6) Zammit, A. R., Robitaille, A., Piccinin, A. M., Muniz-Terrera, G., & Hofer, S. M. (2019). "Associations Between Aging-Related Changes in Grip Strength and Cognitive Function in Older Adults: A Systematic Review." *Journal of Gerontology: Series A, Biological Sciences and Medical Sciences, 74*(4), 519–527. Retrieved from https://pmc.ncbi.nlm.nih.gov/articles/PMC6417444/.
7) Physiopedia. (n.d.). "Guyon Canal Syndrome." *Physiopedia*. Retrieved from https://www.physio-pedia.com/Guyon_Canal_Syndrome.
8) Gorman, K. F., Julien, C., & Moreau, A. (2012). "The Genetic Epidemiology of Idiopathic Scoliosis." *European Spine Journal*, 21(10), 1905–1919. doi:10.1007/s00586-012-2389-6. Retrieved from https://doi.org/10.1007/s00586-012-2389-6
9) "Hernia: A Common Problem for Men with Age." MUSC Health. Retrieved from https://advance.muschealth.org/library/2021/july/hernia.
10) Ergomat. (n.d.). "A Summary of Ergonomic Studies of Anti-fatigue Mats." *Ergomat International*. Retrieved from https://intl.ergomat.com/PDF/ergonomic_studies/A-Summary-of-Ergonomic-Studies-of-Anti-fatigue-Mats.pdf.
11) Clancy, K. (2010). "Comparison of Lumbar Spine Loads During Back and Front Squats." *Master's Theses*, State University of New York College at Cortland. Retrieved from https://digitalcommons.cortland.edu/theses/86/

12) Caring Medical. (n.d.). "Torn Hip Labrum: Repair and Prolotherapy." *Caring Medical Regenerative Medicine Clinics*. Retrieved from https://caringmedical.com/prolotherapy-news/torn-hip-labrum-repair-prolotherapy/.
13) An updated review of femoroacetabular impingement syndrome. Orthopedic Reviews. https://doi.org/10.52965/001c.37513
14) Kapron AL, Anderson AE, Aoki SK, Phillips LG, Petron DJ, Toth R, Peters CL. Radiographic prevalence of femoroacetabular impingement in collegiate football players: AAOS Exhibit Selection. J Bone Joint Surg Am. 2011 Oct 5;93(19):e111(1-10). doi: 10.2106/JBJS.K.00544. PMID: 22005872.
15) Frank, J. M., Harris, J. D., Erickson, B. J., Slikker, W., 3rd, Bush-Joseph, C. A., Salata, M. J., & Nho, S. J. (2015). Prevalence of Femoroacetabular Impingement Imaging Findings in Asymptomatic Volunteers: A Systematic Review. *Arthroscopy : the journal of arthroscopic & related surgery : official publication of the Arthroscopy Association of North America and the International Arthroscopy Association*, 31(6), 1199–1204. https://doi.org/10.1016/j.arthro.2014.11.042
16) Occupational Safety and Health Administration (OSHA). (n.d.). "Ergonomics: The Study of Work." *U.S. Department of Labor*. Retrieved from https://www.osha.gov/ergonomics.
17) American Academy of Orthopaedic Surgeons. (2022). "One in Two Americans Have a Musculoskeletal Condition." *ScienceDaily*. Retrieved from https://www.sciencedaily.com/releases/2016/03/160301114116.htm.

18) Culvenor, A. G., Collins, N. J., Guermazi, A., Cook, J. L., & Vicenzino, B. (2019). *Prevalence of knee osteoarthritis features on magnetic resonance imaging in asymptomatic uninjured adults: A systematic review and meta-analysis*. British Journal of Sports Medicine, 53(20), 1268–1278.
https://doi.org/10.1136/bjsports-2018-099257
19) Horga, L.M., Hirschmann, A.C., Henckel, J. et al. Prevalence of abnormal findings in 230 knees of asymptomatic adults using 3.0 T MRI. *Skeletal Radiol* 49, 1099–1107 (2020).
https://doi.org/10.1007/s00256-020-03394-z
20) Mayo Clinic Staff. (2023). "Knee bursitis - Symptoms and causes." *Mayo Clinic*. Retrieved from https://www.mayoclinic.org/diseases-conditions/knee-bursitis/symptoms-causes/syc-20355501.
21) Smith, J. D., et al. (2019). "The Effect of Sleep Position on Joint Pain and Spine Health: A Systematic Review." *Clinical Orthopaedics and Related Research*, 477(3), 537–545. doi:10.1097/CORR.0000000000000621. Retrieved from https://doi.org/10.1097/CORR.0000000000000621.
22) Atherton, A. (2021). "3 Steps to Building Your Calf Strength." *Runner's World UK*. Retrieved from https://www.runnersworld.com/uk/health/injury/a775672/3-steps-to-building-your-calf-strength/.

About Us
Dr. Ariana Fontenot
Doctor of Physical Therapy

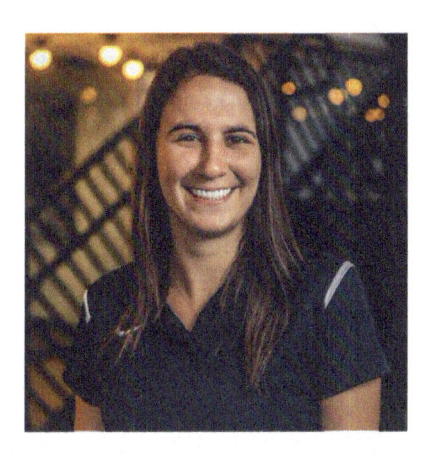

I grew up in a family of doctors — my mom is an Infectious Disease Specialist. Surrounded by medicine, I naturally gravitated toward healthcare—but my heart belonged to sports. I was passionate about soccer, playing on teams that won three state titles, and I dreamed of becoming an orthopedic surgeon so I could stay connected to the sports world forever.

That plan took a turn after I sustained a knee injury that required surgery. I went to the best surgeon around, confident I was on the right path. But after the operation, something shifted. I realized I didn't just care about the procedure—I cared about what came after: the recovery, the process of rebuilding. I couldn't imagine being the person who operated and then walked away, never seeing how the story ended.

During my rehab, my physical therapists motivated me, but there was one problem: I never did a single home exercise. They were too complicated, too easy to skip, and, frankly, they didn't stick. Ever since, I've been committed to implementing exercises that are so easy they feel automatic and you can do them anywhere.

What's simpler than exercises? Habits. Instead of adding more to your to-do list, I focus on turning the things you're already doing into opportunities for movement and healing. It's not about working harder; it's about working smarter.

Encouraged by my patients, whose lives were transformed by the Slight Motion Method, I felt inspired to share their stories and spread the word to help others. Their successes motivated me to write this book and bring the Slight Motion Method to a broader audience. Inspired by the mission to *"change the world one person at a time"* I'm dedicated to making pain-free living accessible to everyone.

Today, as a Doctor of Physical Therapy, I live to motivate people — not just to recover, but to thrive. The principle *"A little goes a long way,"* isn't just a slogan; it's the heartbeat of everything I do. Healing doesn't start with a complicated routine. It starts with awareness. It starts with a single habit.

Dr. Marla Lester
Doctor of Physical Therapy

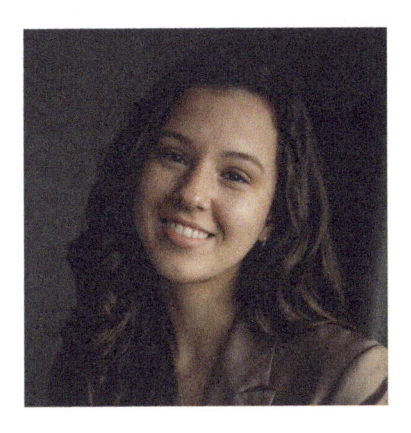

Dr. Marla Lester grew up in sunny South Florida, inspired by a lifelong passion for movement, health, and helping others live pain-free lives. As a former athlete, she experienced the impact of injury and recovery firsthand. Her journey into physical therapy was fueled by a deep curiosity about how the human body works and a commitment to finding solutions that truly make a difference.

As a Doctor of Physical Therapy and co-founder of Slight Motion PT, Marla has dedicated her career to uncovering the hidden connections between daily habits and chronic pain.
Specializing in manual therapy and dry needling, she blends anatomy and skill to deliver transformative care. Marla's approach is grounded in the belief that pain isn't just a symptom to treat—it's a signal to decode.

She works closely with clients to identify the movements, positions, and patterns contributing to their discomfort, creating personalized solutions that are simple, actionable, and incredibly effective.

Her work is fueled by years of hands-on experience and collaboration with the top experts in the field, always seeking new ways to help people move better and feel better. Through education and strategic interventions, she empowers people to not just recover, but to thrive.

"We're not just treating pain," Marla says. "We're teaching people how to move through life differently so they can feel better every day."

Testimonials

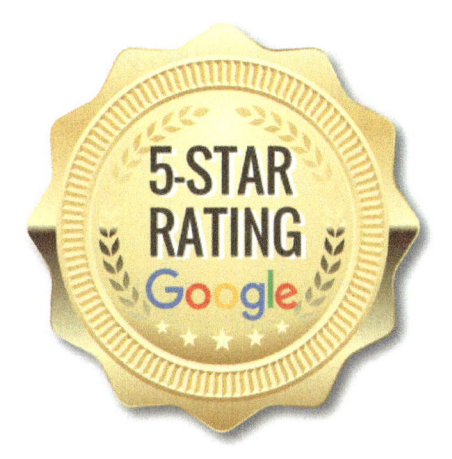

"I'm 60 and I've been struggling with intermittent sciatic pain. I've tried chiropractors and Aleve to no avail. The pain had gotten so bad I was unable to walk or play golf. A friend suggested I see Ariana. I started receiving treatment and within two weeks the pain was minimized. I credit Ariana with a viable treatment plan and therapy guidelines. The next step I'm taking with her is strengthening exercises to protect my hip, back and core. If you're feeling like your quality of life is diminished, schedule an appointment today. I don't know why anyone would want to feel bad when there are people like Ariana in the world."

"Marla is AMAZING. She is a consummate and talented professional, incredibly perceptive, a great listener and motivator. She created a solid plan, taught me the appropriate exercises and helped me to incorporate my daily routines into this journey. She's the best!"

"Dr. Ari is a magician. She fixed 4 years of pain in a single session. This might sound like a fake review. It is not! I have seen several doctors and physiotherapists. They have all done things to help relieve the pain temporarily. But Dr. Ari got to the root cause of the issue immediately. And just one lifestyle change resulted in a pain reduction of over 80%. I could wake up with no pain in my back and I felt like a new person."

"I did an ergonomic assessment with Dr. Ariana, which enabled me to learn so much in an hour about how our body works and how the smallest of changes can make or break it. Her expertise and research in this area is unmatched. Her way of teaching is so intuitive that it's actually easy to internalize it and turn it into habits. I can't recommend her enough. She also went out of the way to help with some advice for my mom's knees - how sweet :)"

"I had ACL surgery and started PT at a different clinic before seeing Marla. Best decision I made for recovery. Marla was there for me every step of the way. She was my educator, therapist and cheerleader. I am back to normal activities because of her!"

"Team at Slight Motion will highlight every major factor in improving your posture in a session. Which turns out - are mostly simple things. Highly recommend them!"

"Was experiencing persistent tennis elbow and in one session was able to point out easy daily habit fixes which I didn't even realize were connected to the issue! First time going through cupping and dry needling therapy and I can say one session felt like 10 at any other physical therapist."

"Dr. Marla is amazing and her hands are magical! I've been struggling with back and neck pain and she's helped me with this and more. I've done both cupping and dry needling and I've seen a huge improvement with the pain to the point that I feel almost back to normal. Great patient care, very kind and super knowledgeable. Her expertise is like no other and the combination of her hands, techniques, and post care have made a difference in my life. Thank you Dr. Marla!"

"I've had 2 sessions with Dr. Ariana Fontenot and it's literally changed my life. The wealth of knowledge she shares is unbelievable. I'm sleeping better, using my knees when I was previously afraid but most importantly my bunions are correcting themselves and for the first time in months I don't have toe pain! Thank you, I can't wait to read your book and I've told all my friends!"

"Marla is the best!!!! Whether it's my knee, my neck, my back, or even my jaw, Marla uses her expertise and incredible technique to fix me right up. I recently had a dry-needling session with her to relieve my neck pain. I tend to be sensitive to hands-on therapy but needling has changed the game for me. I will definitely be booking more sessions!
Thanks Dr. Marla!"

"After many other physiotherapy sessions leaving me feeling discouraged because of the unrealistic need of maintaining specific postural positions and practices, Dr. Ariana Fontenot changed my entire view on what best practices look like. She led my session by showing me small adjustments I can make without changing my routines - making the entire process much more approachable and realistic and showing me how the most minute changes can positively affect my overall body comfortability."

"Ariana came over and helped me out with my 4 year old neck injury. Went through my daily routine to help correct what I was habitually doing wrong such as sleep/couch posture and how I sit in my car. Released tension, showed me exercises and is improving. Real nice, professional gal. Look forward to the next session!"

"Marla is an excellent therapist. With her program she's improved my mobility to the extent that I have not felt this good in years."

"Ariana is very knowledgeable about what causes pain, and ways to fix it in your everyday life. I was having bad knee pain and she taught me ways to fix it in my everyday life, that are actually reasonable. She likes to fix pain from the source which is super important. She also has texted me multiple times following up with how I am doing, and takes the time to listen to her patients. The amount of care I have seen from her is more than anyone I could find."

Made in the USA
Coppell, TX
24 February 2025